THE DIALYSIS HANDBOOK
FOR TECHNICIANS AND NURSES

2nd Edition

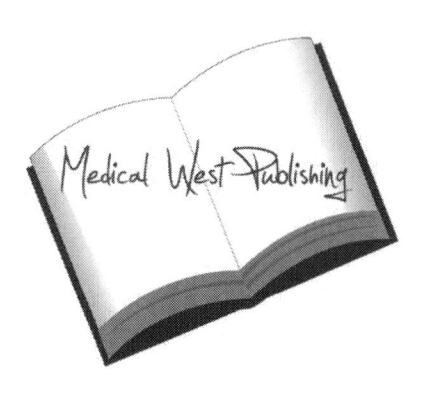

Medical West Publishing

Medical West Publishing

© Copyright 2012
P.O. Box 22
West Covina, CA. 91793

All rights reserved. No part of this book may be reproduced in any form or by any means, including information storage and retrieval systems, without permission in writing from the publisher, except by a reviewer who my quote brief passages in a review.

THE DIALYSIS HANDBOOK
FOR TECHNICIANS AND NURSES

Oscar M. Cairoli, BSN, MA, RN, PHN

Senior Operational Consultant
Renal Business Group
Kaiser Permanente
Pasadena, CA

Dedicated to my two sons:

Oscar Cairoli, III
Jonathan Cairoli

Contents

Chapter 1 **Components, Functions, Purposes** *Page 11*
Components of the kidney
Components and functions of the nephron
Components of the urinary system
Components of the artificial kidney
Comparative functions of the human and the artificial kidney
Purpose of dialysis

Chapter 2 **Chronic Kidney Disease – CKD** *Page 23*

Chapter 3 **Hemodialysis** *Page 27*

Chapter 4 **Access for Hemodialysis** *Page 31*
External accesses – Arteriovenous shunt
External accesses – Catheters
Internal accesses – A.V. fistula
Internal accesses – Bovine graft
Internal accesses – A.V. graft
Points to remember
Advantages and disadvantages of external vs. internal access – External access
Advantages and disadvantages of external vs. internal access – Internal access

Chapter 5 **Peritoneal Dialysis** *Page 41*

Chapter 6 **Blood Chemistries: Implications for Hemodialysis** *Page 47*
Blood urea nitrogen
Calcium
Chloride
Creatinine
Glucose
Iron
Magnesium
Phosphate
Potassium
Sodium
Uric acid
Normal chemistries

Chapter 7 **Electrolyte Imbalance: Signs and Symptoms** *Page 63*
Calcium deficit – Hypocalcemia
Calcium excess – Hypercalcemia
Magnesium deficit – Hypomagnesemia
Potassium deficit – Hypokalemia
Potassium excess – Hyperkalemia

Sodium deficit – Hyponatremia
Sodium excess – Hypernatremia

Chapter 8   **Potential Problems in Hemodialysis**   *Page 71*
Air embolus
Angina
Arm pain
Bleeding A.V. access
Blood loss
Blood transfusion reaction
Blood vessel spasm
Bone disease
Cardiac dysrhythmias
Clotting in the dialyzer
Cramps
Dyspnea
Eye changes
Fever/Chills
Headache
Hemolysis
Hypertension
Hypotension
Infection
Nausea and vomiting
Neuropathy
Power failure
Pruritus
Seizures

Chapter 9   **Secondary Problems of Renal Failure**   *Page 121*
Cardiovascular
Dermatological
Endocrine
Gastrointestinal
Hemotologic
Metabolic
Neurological
Ocular
Peripheral Neuropathy
Psychological

Chapter 10   **Diagnostic Studies**   *Page 133*
Chest x-ray
Echocardiography
Electrocardiogram
Fistulagram
Metabolic bone survey
Nerve conduction study

Chapter 11 **Dialysates, Dialyzers** *Page 141*
Composition of dialyzing fluid
Components of the dialyzer
Coil
Hoeltzenbeim
Hollow fiber
Parallel or flat plate

Chapter 12 **Hemodialysis Equipment and Water Treatment** *Page 149*
Air detector
Batch delivery system
Bed-side station
Blood pump
Central delivery system
Heparin pump
Proportioning unit – single patient
Single-needle device
Sorbsystem
Water treatment

Chapter 13 **Renal Case Management** *Page 161*

Chapter 14 **History** *Page 165*

Chapter 15 **Dialysis Acronyms** *Page 169*

Appendices *Page 231*
Access options – Pros and cons
Table of commonly used equivalent values
Viral hepatitis overview
Liver function tests
Formulas
Essential terms of direction and movement
Related web sites

References *Page 242*

Suggestions *Page 243*

Practice Questions *Page 244*

Preface

The Dialysis Handbook for Technicians and Nurses was created to meet a need for the health care giver in dialysis, whether an RN, a LVN/LPN, or a patient care technician.

In the **Second Edition**, it was expanded with information regarding Peritoneal Dialysis, and Chronic Kidney Disease (CKD), as other information related to this field. Also the art work was re-done and new drawings were added.

For the person just entering this complex field, **The Dialysis Handbook for Technicians and Nurses** provides an organized approach to the immense amount of data that must be learned; for the experienced person in dialysis, this book fills the need for quick, on-the-spot reference. **The Dialysis Handbook for Technicians and Nurses** is a reference that includes data on high-priority areas. I recommend you consult basic medical-surgical, nephrology, and pharmaceutical texts for more detailed information.

While I have outlined each chapter according to our practice, the contents of **The Dialysis Handbook for Technicians and Nurses** are not to be construed as standing orders for treatment. Each dialysis facility has its own guidelines, policies, and protocols, dictated in part by the laws governing their state of residence; I refer you to these.

Some specific information on this book reflects medical equipment or procedures no longer in use but they have historical importance in this field, this information will be noted as *historical*.

I like to acknowledge the help and support that have been extended to me during the years by dedicated technicians, nurses, physicians, and other members of the renal team. And my deepest appreciation goes to the **dialysis patient** who has giving me the reason to be a nephrology nurse for over 30 years. And last but not least, I like to express my gratitude to Myrna Barrios-Craig for her support during this project.

Art work was done by:
Michele Graham, MS MFA
Board Certified Medical Illustrator & Fine Artist
email: mgstudios@q.com

TO THE STUDENT/READER

This is a working book, feel free to write your own notes, ideas, questions in the spaces provided for you. Take this book with you to the clinical area and use it as a reference.

Chapter 1

Components, Functions, Purposes

Components of the Kidney

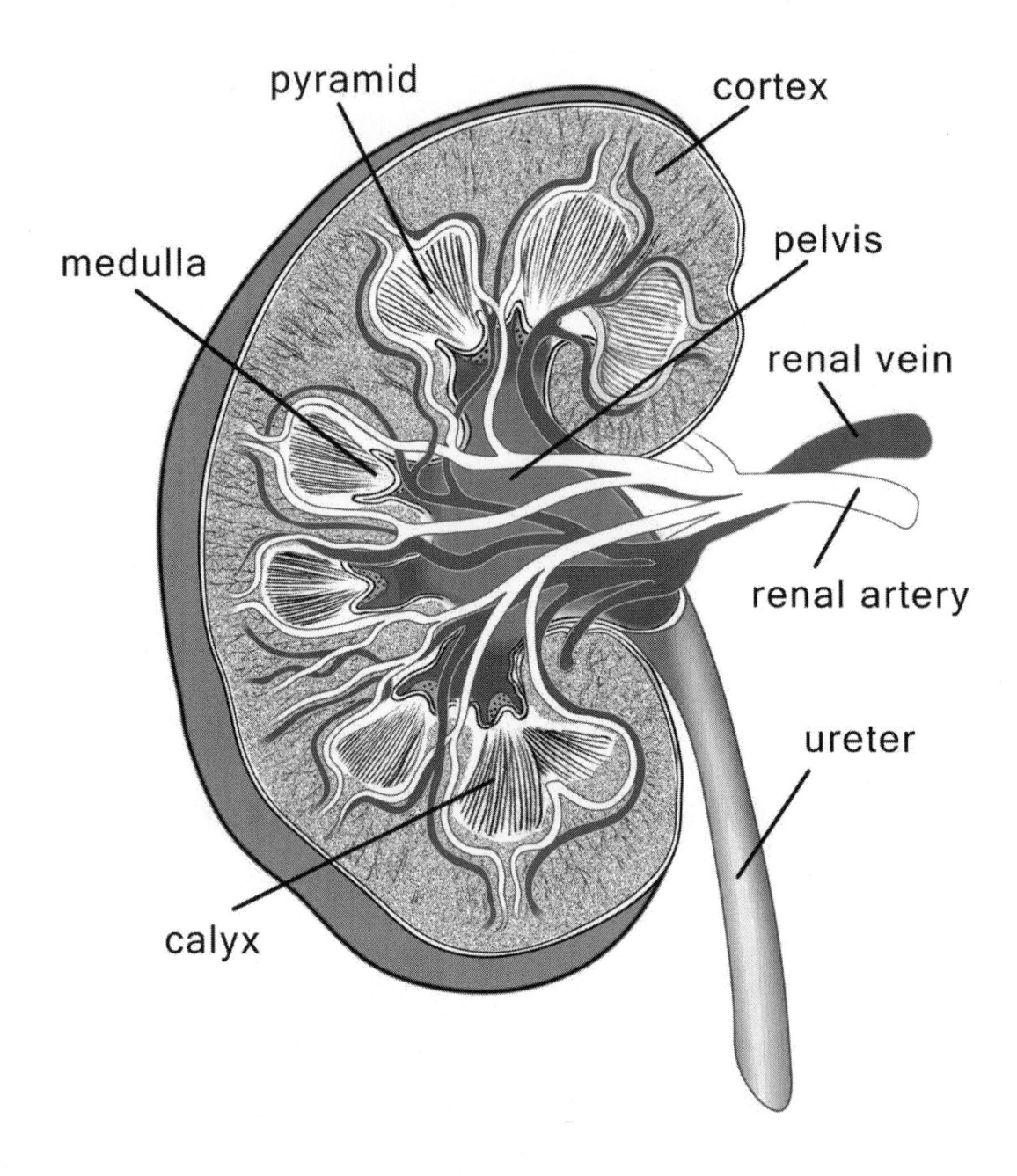

Figure 1

Components of the Kidney

Figure 1

a. Cortex	Contains the blood vessels and branches called glomeruli.
b. Medulla	Contains the collecting tubules.
c. Pyramid	Contains the collecting apparatus and the tubules.
d. Calyx	Is the cuplike division of the kidney pelvis.
e. Renal Artery	Supplies the blood to the kidney.
f. Renal Vein	Evacuates the blood from the kidney.
g. Pelvis	Collects the urine.
h. Ureters	Convey the urine from the kidney to the bladder.

Components and Functions of the Nephron

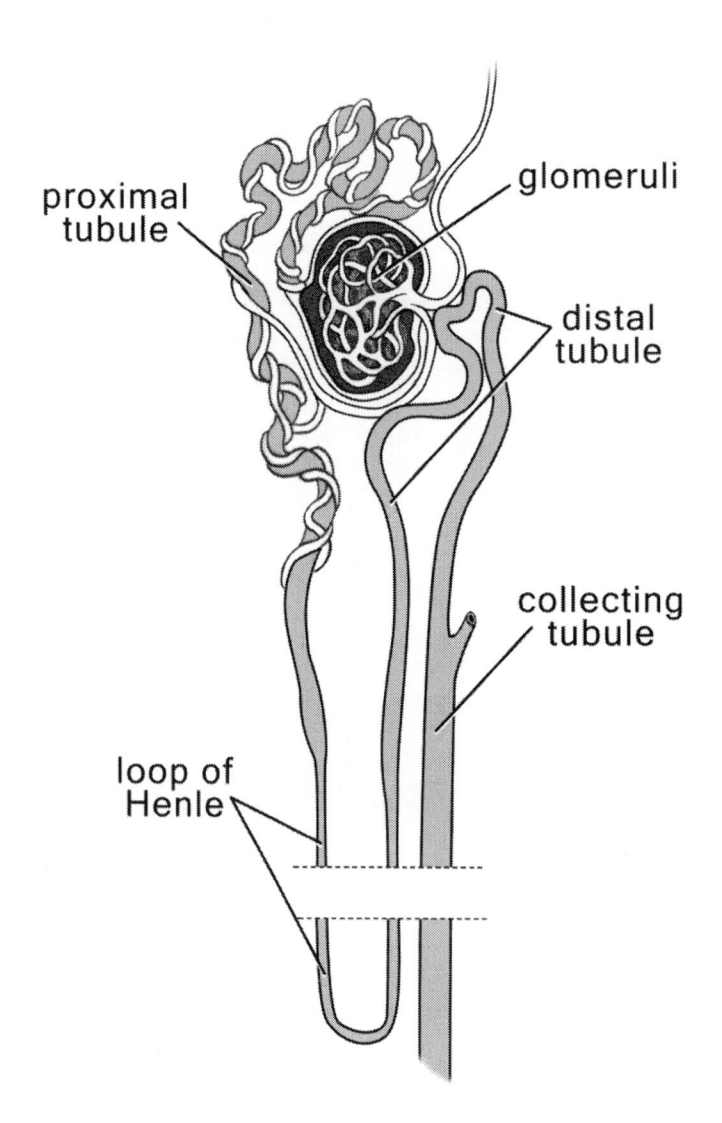

Figure 2

Components and Functions of the Nephron

Figure 2

Part of Nephron	Function	Substance
a. Glomeruli	Filtration	H2O and solute, electrolytes, urea, Creatinine, uric acid, glucose, amino acids.
b. Proximal tubules	Reabsorption, secretion	H2O, electrolytes, glucose, amino acids.
c. Loop of Henle	Reabsorption	H2O, electrolytes (Na, K).
d. Distal tubule	Acid-base balance, secretion	Hydrogen ions (H), Na.
e. Collecting tubule	Concentration	H2O.

Components of the Urinary System

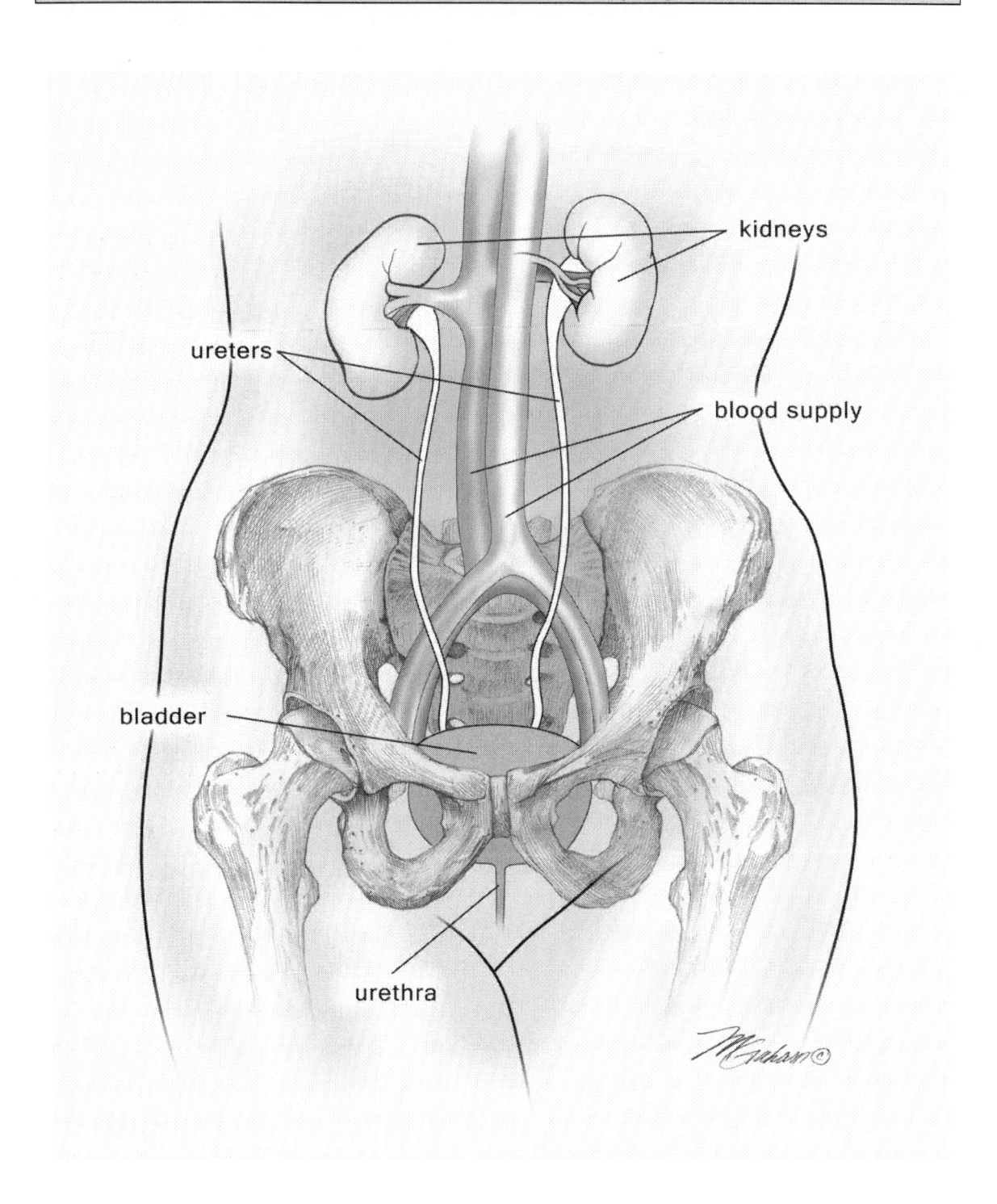

Figure 3

Components of the Urinary System

Figure 3

a. **Blood supply** - Every day, a person's kidneys process about 200 quarts of blood to sift out about 2 quarts of waste products and extra water.

b. **Kidneys** - The kidneys are bean-shaped organs, each about the size of a fist. They are located near the middle of the back, just below the rib cage, one on each side of the spine. The kidneys are sophisticated reprocessing machines.

c. **Ureters** - The wastes and extra water become urine, which flows to the bladder through tubes called ureters.

d. **Bladder** - The bladder stores urine until releasing it through urination.

e. **Urethra** – It is a tube that connects the urinary bladder to the genitals for the removal of fluids out of the body.

Components of the Artificial Kidney

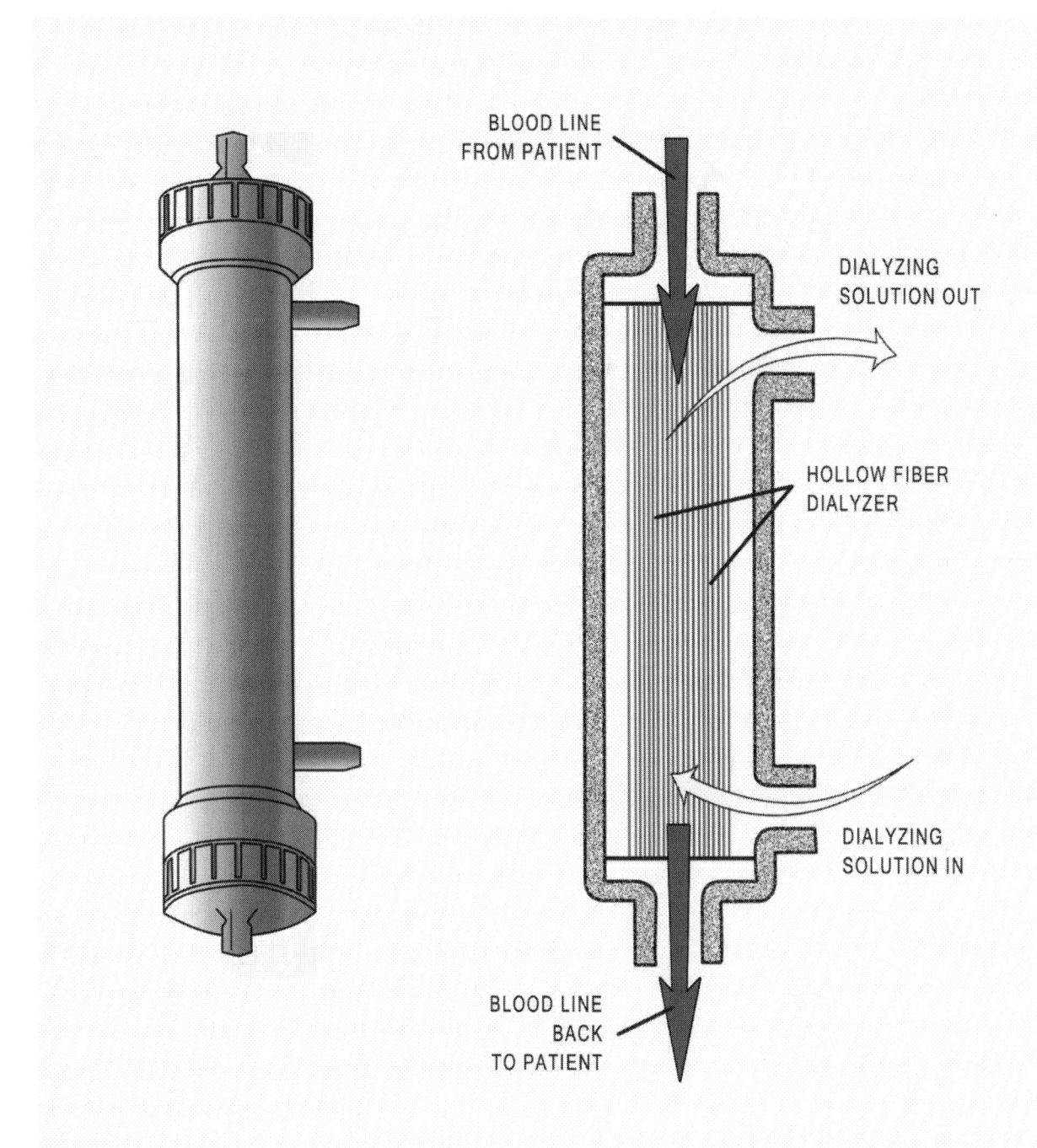

Figure 4

Components of the Artificial Kidney

Figure 4

a. Blood lines (blood supply)

b. Dialyzer (kidneys)

c. Dialysate lines (ureters, bladder, urethra)

Comparative Functions of the Human and the Artificial Kidney

The Human Kidney

    a. Excretes waste.
    b. Adjusts composition of body fluids.
    c. Excretes and detoxifies drugs.
    d. Provides intermediary metabolism
- Vitamin D
- Insulin, glucose

    e. Provides endocrine functions
- Produces renin
- Produces erythropoietin

The Artificial Kidney (Dialyzer)

    a. Excretes water-soluble waste products or those broken down as a water-soluble product.
    b. Adjusts composition of body fluids.
    c. Removes some drugs.

Purpose of Dialysis

To remove metabolic wastes, other poisons, and excess fluids from the body by artificial means when the natural kidney function is inadequate (as in End Stage Renal Disease, acute renal failure, drug overdose).

This is accomplished primarily by osmosis, the passage of solvent through a semipermeable membrane, using a dialyzer (hemodialysis), or the peritoneal membrane (peritoneal dialysis or PD) from a solution of lower concentration of solute to one of higher concentration.

NOTES

If you can dream it,
You can do it.

-Walt Disney

Chapter 2

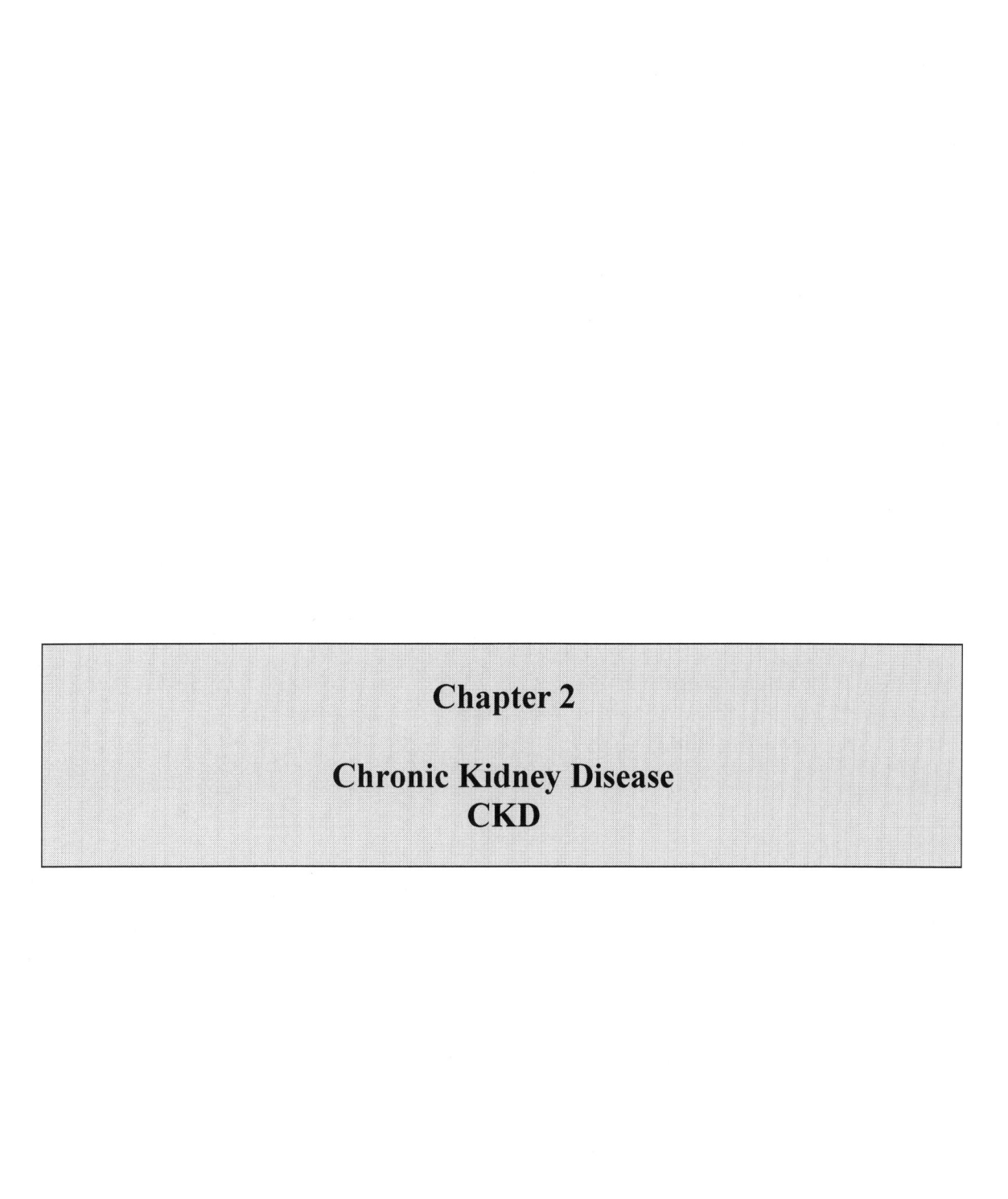

Chronic Kidney Disease
CKD

Chronic Kidney Disease - CKD

Stages of CKD – The National Kidney Foundation's Kidney Disease Outcome Quality Initiative (KDOQI) has suggested staging CKD from stage 1 (mildest) to stage 5 (most severe) based on the level of estimated glomerular filtration rate or GFR normalized to body surface area.

CKD Stages

Stage	Description	GFR
1	Kidney damage with normal or supranormal GFR	≥ 90
2	Kidney damage with mild decrease in GFR	60-89
3	Moderate decrease in GFR	30-69
4	Severe decrease in GFR	15-29
5	Kidney failure	<15

Treatment Choices

Choices - The patient and family should have proper education of their options for treatment. Usually is called: "The Choices Class."

The options – We have basically four options that the patient with CKD can choose from when treatment is needed. The four options are as follows:

- Hemodialysis
- Peritoneal dialysis
- Transplant
- No treatment

NOTES

The important thing is not to stop questioning.

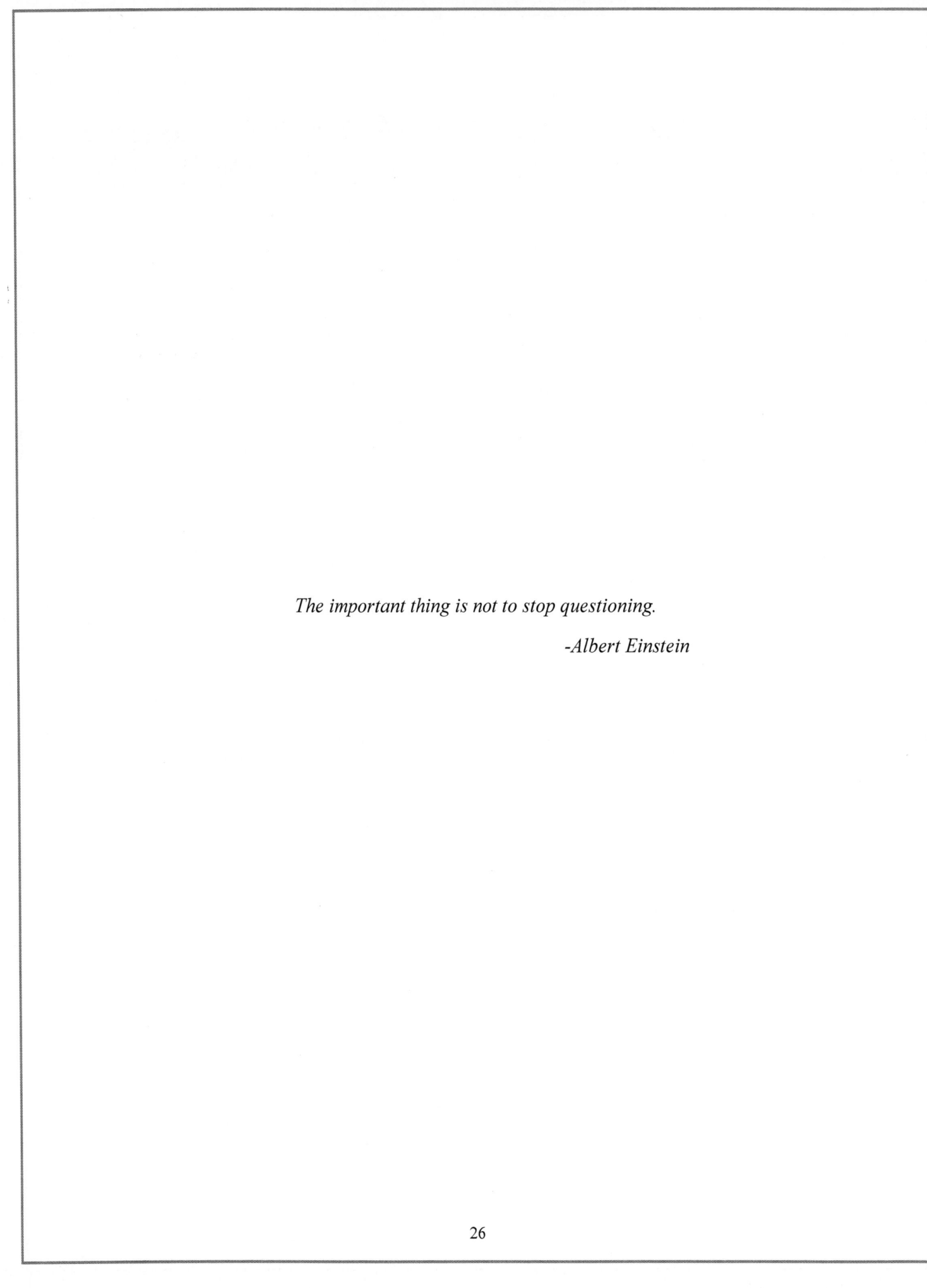

-Albert Einstein

Chapter 3
Hemodialysis

Hemodialysis

Conventional Hemodialysis

Chronic hemodialysis is usually done three times per week, for about 3-4 hours for each treatment, during which the patient's blood is drawn out through a tube at a rate of 300-400 cc/min. The tube is connected to a 15, 16, or 17 gauge needle inserted in the dialysis fistula or graft, or connected to one port of a dialysis catheter. The blood is then pumped through the dialyser (filter), and then the processed blood is pumped back into the patient's bloodstream through another tube (connected to a second needle or port). During the procedure, the patient's blood pressure is closely monitored, and if it becomes low, or the patient develops any other signs of low blood volume such as nausea, the dialysis attendant can administer extra fluid through the machine. During the treatment, the patient's entire blood volume (about 5000 cc) circulates through the machine every 15 minutes.

Daily Hemodialysis

Daily hemodialysis is typically used by those patients who do their own dialysis at home. It is less stressful (more gentle) but does require more frequent access. This is simple with catheters, but more problematic with fistulas or grafts. The "buttonhole technique" can be used for fistulas requiring frequent access. Daily hemodialysis is usually done for 2 hours six days a week. This modality is usually done at home.

Nocturnal Hemodialysis

The procedure of nocturnal hemodialysis is similar to conventional hemodialysis except it is performed six nights a week and six-ten hours per session while the patient sleeps. It can be done at home or in some dialysis centers where they offer this modality.

Hemodialysis

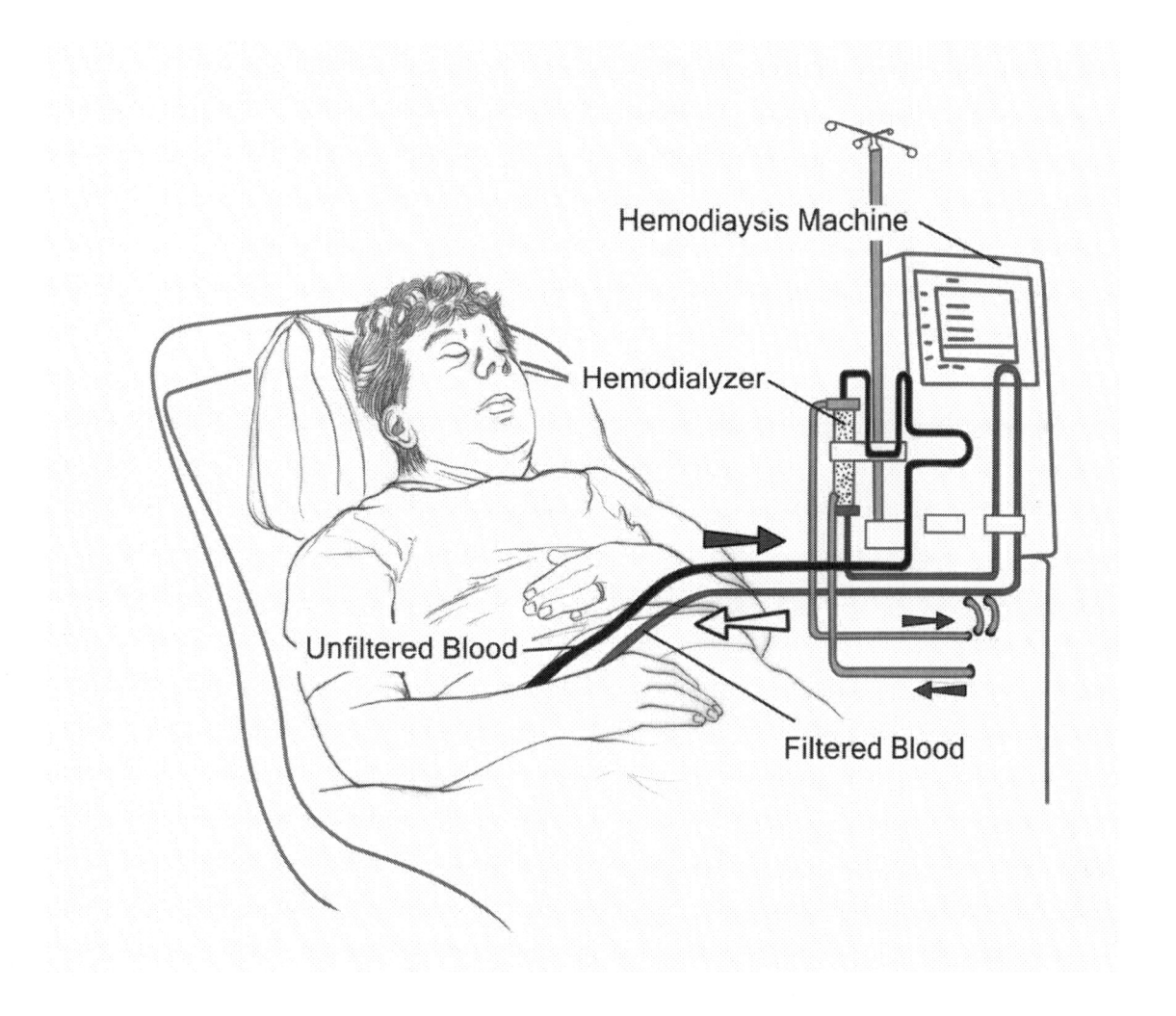

Figure 5

NOTES

*If we all did the things we are capable of,
we would astound ourselves.*

- Thomas Edison

Chapter 4

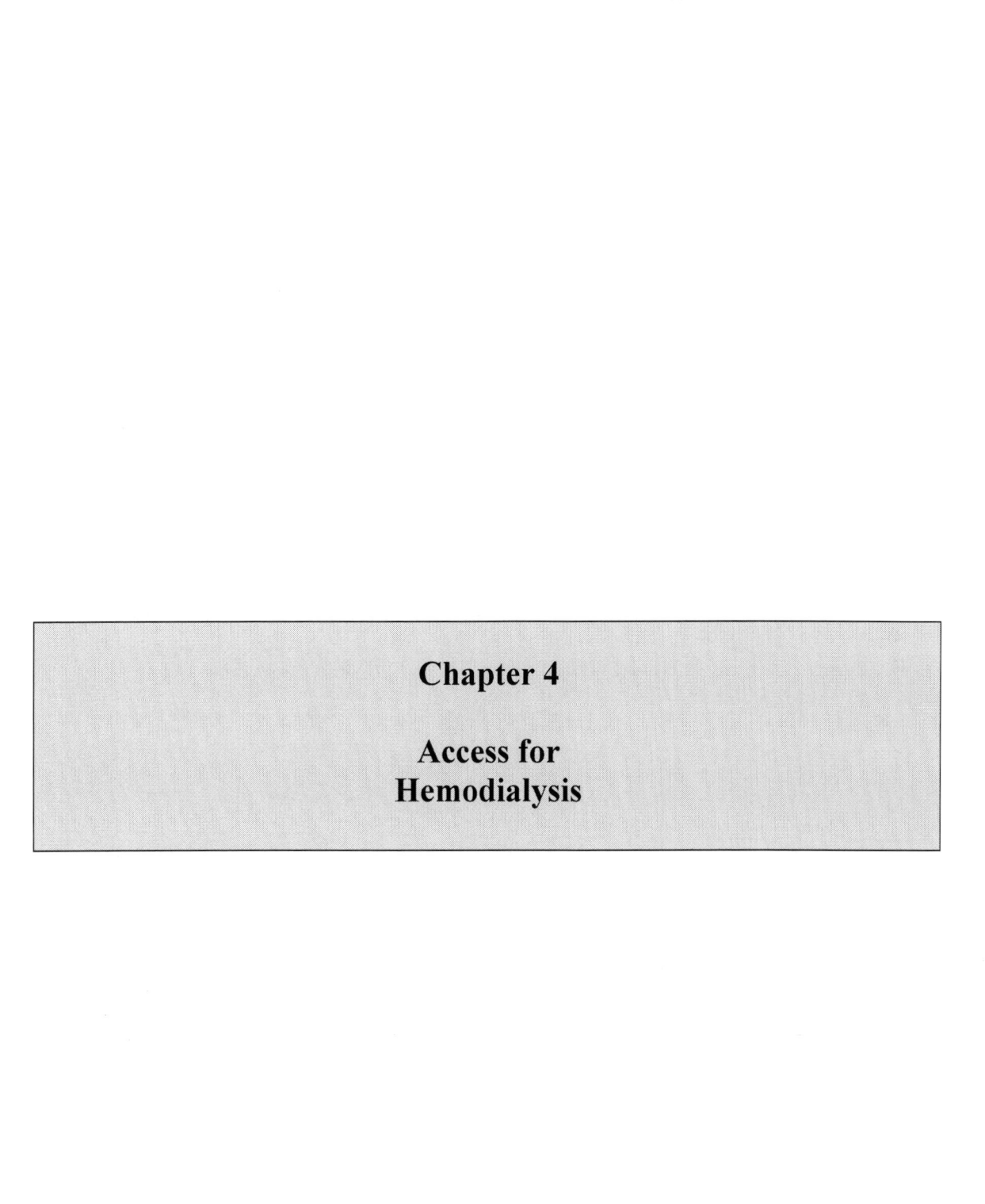

Access for Hemodialysis

External Accesses

Arteriovenous Shunt — HISTORICAL

"To shunt," means to shift or divert. An arteriovenous shunt is a device that diverts blood flow by an external pathway from artery to a vein. Dialysis personnel speak of a *shunt* or a *cannula*; the terms are interchangeable. A cannula is a tube for insertion into a body cavity or blood vessel; when inserted into an artery and vein, it is then commonly known as an *arteriovenous (AV) shunt.* A short length of the cannula, about 1-½ inches, lies directly within the host blood vessel. The cannula tip is held in place with a surgical tie or ligature.

The AV shunt requires meticulous care. Successful hemodialysis depends upon a clean, healthy shunt. Proper shunt care is not difficult, but it does require a certain amount of attention.

Dr. Belding Scribner described the shunt in 1960. This Teflon cannula was typically placed in the radial artery with return through the cephalic vein.

NOTES

Catheters

Temporary angioaccess is frequently required in the setting of acute renal failure, acute intoxications, and in the ESRD patient who may lose their chronic dialysis access to thrombosis or infection. This access to the circulation is most often furnished by coaxial dual-lumen vascular catheters. To minimize recirculation the venous and arterial ports are spaced 2 to 3 cm apart.

These catheters are usually inserted at the bedside. For relatively short-term treatments the femoral vein is the site of choice.

Cuffed tunnel catheters have come into long-term use for patients without viable peripheral vascular access. The design of these devices has increased their use beyond that of acute catheters. Improved survival on hemodialysis has increased the number of patients without peripheral access and thus has increased the use of these catheters. I addition, initiation of dialysis in an older, diabetic population prone to peripheral vascular disease has likewise increased our reliance on cuffed catheters.

These catheters (cuffed tunnel) are typically placed with ultrasound guidance to aid insertion, using fluoroscopy to ensure appropriate catheter tip placement. Blood flow rates of 400 ml/min are achievable with some catheter designs, but low blood flow rates due to catheter malfunction are frequent.

NOTES

Internal Accesses

AV Fistula

Created by the anastomosis of a vein and an artery in one of the extremities, usually the lower arm, a fistula is used to provide access for large bore (usually 15, 16, or 17) gauge needles.

After surgery, a healing period is needed, preferably several weeks; exact time will be determined by the vascular surgeon. During the healing phase, the patient will be instructed to do exercises (to develop the vessels) that have been prescribed by the surgeon. These often include applying a tourniquet to the extremity for 5-15 minutes 2-4 times per day (being careful not to cut off circulation completely) and squeezing a rubber ball. This creates pressure within the walls of the vessel, thereby strengthening the walls. Warm, not hot, compresses can also be applied to the area to improve circulation during the exercise period.

When the access is used, prep carefully prior to cannulation to prevent infection (Alcohol should not be used in prepping the access as it is not an effective antimicrobial agent and after long-term use, the skin in the area may become very tough and difficult to cannulate).

NOTES

Bovine Graft

A section of a vessel from a cow is used after it has been treated to avoid any contamination. The vessel is implanted with one end in an artery and the other in a vein.

At least one to two weeks should elapse between surgery and actual use of the graft, when possible; this will be determined by the vascular surgeon.

Use this type of access is the same as the use of a fistula. Be careful not to apply too much pressure on the graft after dialysis is completed in order to prevent unnecessary clot formation in the graft. As with the fistula, prep carefully prior to the use of the access, to prevent infection.

NOTES

AV Graft

A synthetic tube used in place of a bovine graft or AV fistula, it is placed in the same manner as the bovine graft: that is, one end of the tube is attached to an artery and the other to the vein.

Two weeks should elapse between surgery and actual use of the graft when possible (Gore-Tex® or Impra®) for the Vectra® graft it can be used the same day; this will be determined by the vascular surgeon.

Use of this type of access is basically the same as the fistula. Be careful not to apply too much pressure on the graft after dialysis is completed in order to prevent unnecessary clot formation. As with the fistula, prep carefully prior to cannulation of the access to prevent infection.

NOTES

HeRO ™ Vascular Access Device [1]

The HeRO device offers an effective, long-term peripheral access solution for patients who have exhausted peripheral venous access sites suitable for fistulas or grafts. The HeRO device is ideal for patients who:

- Are catheter dependent or are approaching catheter dependency
- Are not candidates for upper extremity AVF or AVG due to poor venous outflow
- Have poor remaining sites for effective creation of AVF or AVG
- Have a failing AVF or AVG due to poor venous outflow
- Have a compromised central venous system
- Are receiving inadequate dialysis clearance via catheters

The HeRO device is completely implanted subcutaneous graft with an outflow component that bypasses central venous stenosis.
Benefits include:

- Significant reduction in bacteremia rates compared to catheters
- Improved adequacy of dialysis and patency with fewer interventions compared to catheters

NOTES

Points to Remember

1. A fistula needs to mature before it can be used (six to eight weeks depending on type).

2. Grafts can be used sooner than a fistula. It is preferable to wait two weeks if possible; this depends on the need to dialyze and the surgeon's preference.

3. The stitches are usually removed two weeks post-surgery.

4. Post-operative, observe for
    a. Patency – presence of bruit or thrill.
    b. Amount of bleeding from the wound site.
    c. Level of pain.
    d. Numbness, tingling, and swelling of the extremity.

5. After the needles are removes, apply pressure to the sites to stop the bleeding. The pressure should be enough to prevent leakage, but not enough to occlude the access.

6. When applying the dressing to clotted access sites, do no create a tourniquet effect. Instruct the patient to check for a pulse at the access site at least three times a day (TID).

NOTES

Advantages and Disadvantages of External vs. Internal Access

External Access

Advantages

1. No needle insertion necessary for dialysis.
2. Access can be used soon after insertion.
3. Blood or lab tests can be drawn without a venipuncture.

Disadvantages

1. Less freedom for the patient.
2. Greater chance for infection.
3. Grater chance of clotting/poor flow, recirculation.
4. Access may become dislodged.

NOTES

Internal Access

Advantages

1. Special precautions unnecessary when working or bathing after healing has occurred.
2. Less chance of infection.
3. Less chance of clotting, recirculation.

Disadvantages

1. Two needle insertions necessary for each dialysis.
2. A large hematoma may form if infiltration occurs.
3. Pressure must be applied post-dialysis when the needles are removed to prevent bleeding (10-30 minutes).

NOTES

Chapter 5

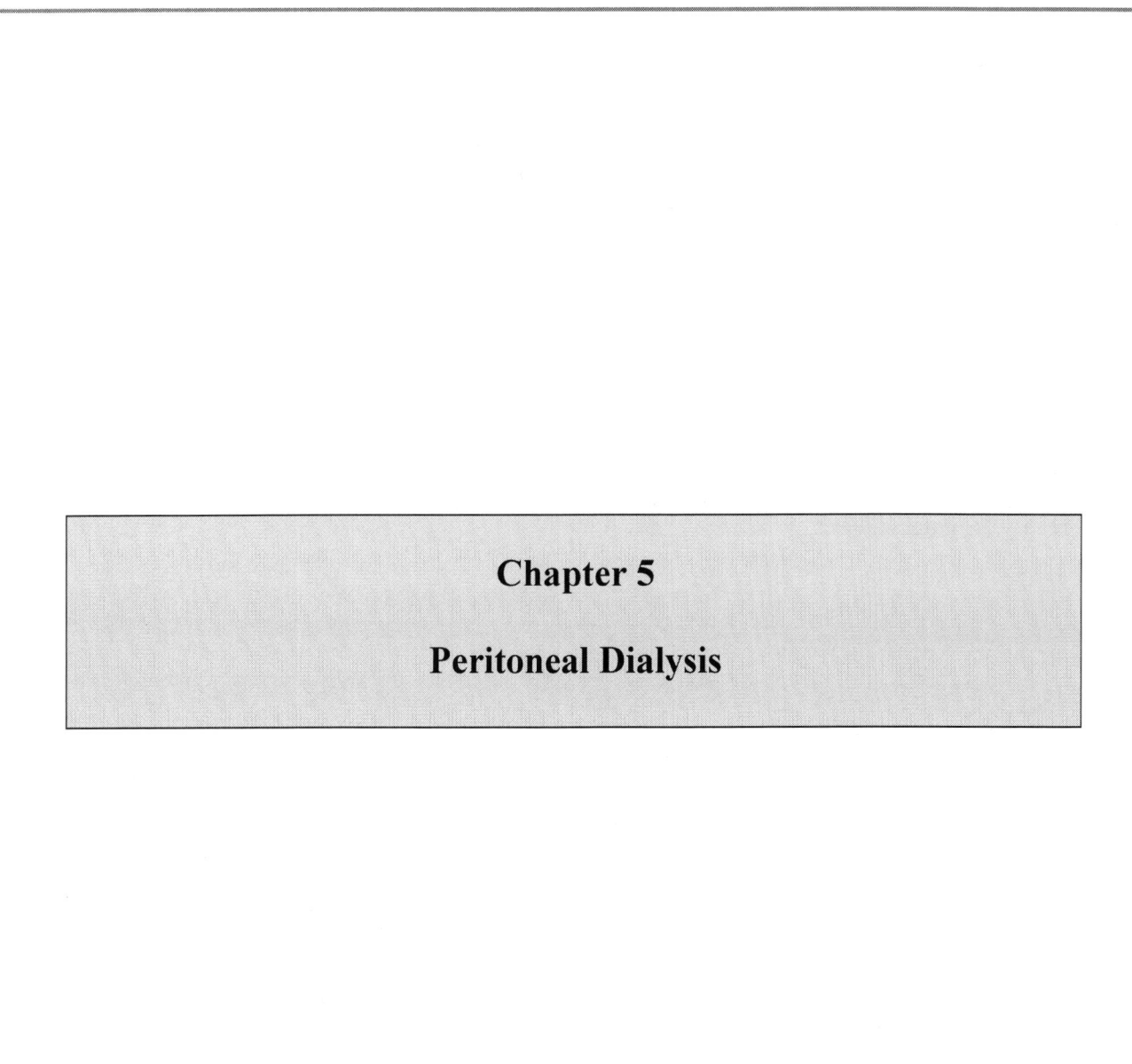

Peritoneal Dialysis

Peritoneal Dialysis

Peritoneal dialysis (PD) is a treatment for patients with severe chronic kidney disease. The process uses the patient's peritoneum in the abdomen as a membrane across which fluids and dissolved substances (electrolytes, urea, glucose, albumin and other small molecules) are exchanged from the blood. Fluid is introduced through a permanent tube in the abdomen and flushed out either every night while the patient sleeps (automatic peritoneal dialysis) or via regular exchanges throughout the day (continuous ambulatory peritoneal dialysis). PD is used as an alternative to hemodialysis though it is far less common. It has comparable risks and expenses, with the primary advantage being the ability to undertake treatment without visiting a medical facility. The primary complication with PD is a risk of infection due to the presence of a permanent tube in the abdomen.

NOTES

Peritoneal Dialysis

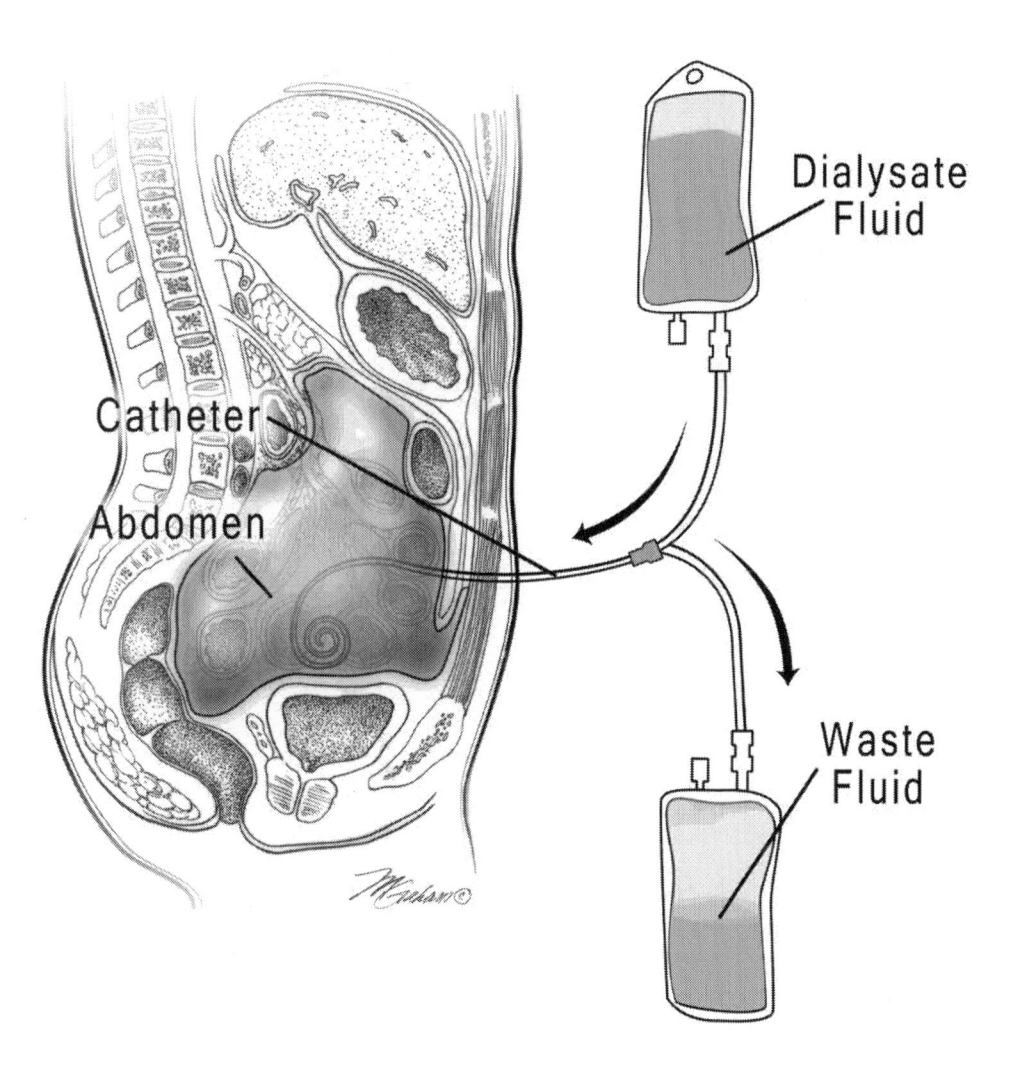

Figure 6

Complications of Peritoneal Dialysis

The main complications of peritoneal dialysis are:

- **Infections.** The most common problem for people receiving peritoneal dialysis is peritonitis, an infection of the abdominal cavity (peritoneum). An infection can also develop at the site where the tube (catheter) is inserted to carry the cleansing fluid into and out of your abdomen.

- **Weight gain.** The fluid used to clean your blood in peritoneal dialysis contains sugar (dextrose). You may take in several hundred calories each day by absorbing some of this fluid, known as dialysate. The extra calories can also lead to high blood sugar if you have diabetes.

- **Weakening of the abdominal muscles (hernia).** Holding fluid in your abdomen for long periods may strain your belly muscles.

NOTES

CAPD vs CCPD

There are different types of peritoneal dialysis:

- **Continuous ambulatory peritoneal dialysis (CAPD).** During CAPD, the dialysate solution stays in your belly for about 4 to 6 hours. After this time, the solution is drained out of your belly. Your belly is then refilled with fresh solution. You need to change the solution about 4 times a day. This is the most commonly used form of peritoneal dialysis.

- **Continuous cycling peritoneal dialysis (CCPD).** During CCPD, a machine automatically fills and drains the dialysate from your belly. This process takes about 10 to 12 hours, so you can perform CCPD at night while you sleep.

NOTES

PD Catheters

The picture below shows different types of PD catheters:

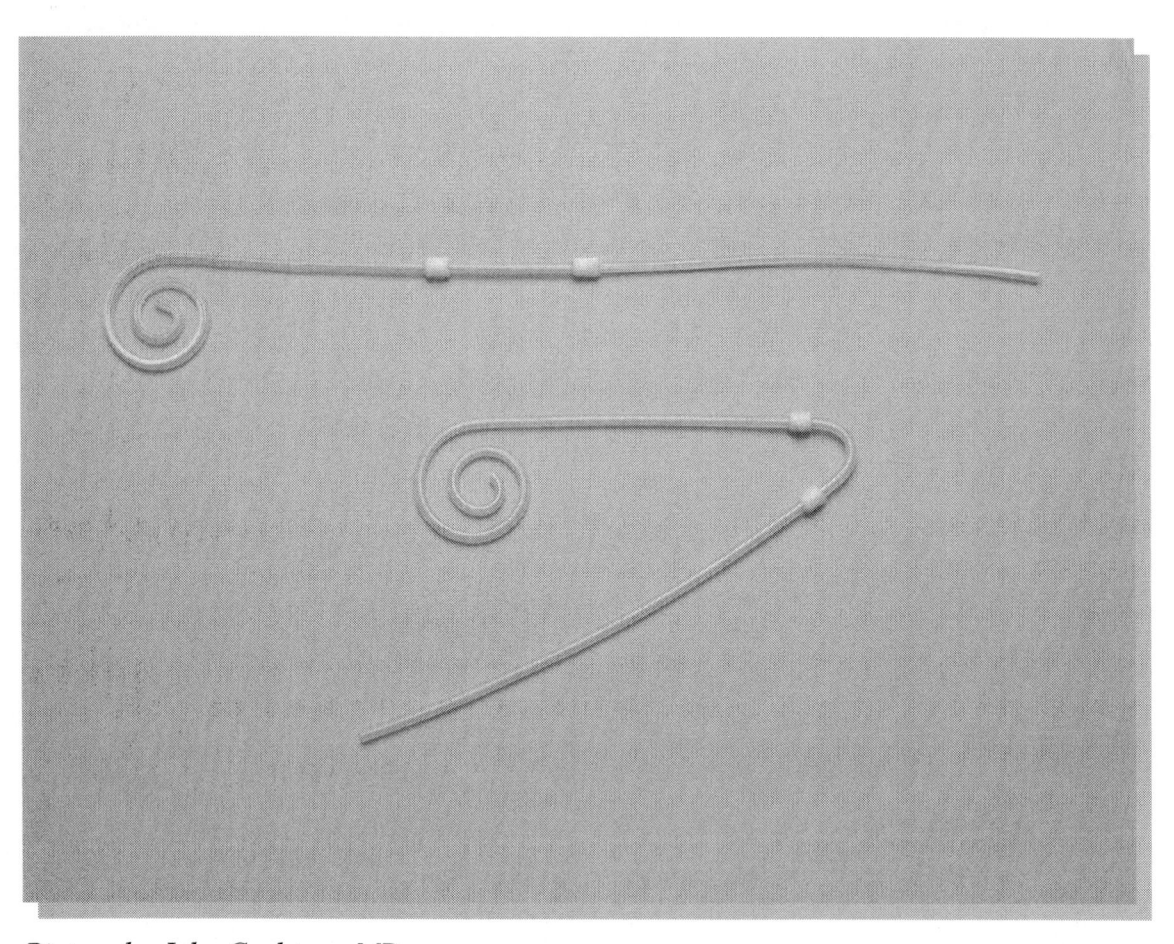

Picture by John Crabtree, MD

Figure 7

NOTES

Chapter 6

**Blood Chemistries:
Indications for Hemodialysis**

*Knowledge is of two kinds:
we know a subject ourselves,
or we know where we can find information on it.*

- Samuel Johnson

Blood Urea Nitrogen (BUN)

Urea is the form in which nitrogen is released from the body. It is the chief nitrogenous constituent of the urine and is the final product of the metabolism of proteins of the body.

Elevated BUN concentration may be the outcome from inadequate renal function (which decreases the rate of urea removal), from excess protein ingestion, or from cellular protein catabolism. Sepsis, gastrointestinal bleeding, and certain antibodies may also increase the BUN levels in the blood.

Normal level: 6-25 mg/dl

NOTES

During dialysis, Pre and Post BUNs are done to check the quality of the treatment. (URR or Urea Reduction Ratio).

Calcium

Calcium is the most abundant mineral in the body. In combination with phosphorus, it forms calcium phosphate, the dense hard materials of the bones and teeth. A constant level of a small amount of calcium in the blood is required for certain important body functions, including maintenance of the heart beat, clotting of the blood, and normal functioning of muscles and nerves.

One half of the circulating calcium exists as the physiologically active free calcium ion; the rest is bound to protein.

When calcium blood levels fall, the parathyroid hormone releases calcium salts from the bone. Any excess calcium will be excreted in the urine by the normal kidneys.

Hemodialysis does not correct the disordered calcium-phosphorus metabolism, and progressive osteodystrophy is a serious problem for many chronic hemodialysis patients.

Calcium can be added to the dialysate to compensate for a decreased level in the serum.

Normal level: 8.5-10.5 mg/dl

NOTES

Dietary sources of calcium include dairy products such as milk and cheese, which are the readiest sources of the mineral.

Chloride

A salt of hydrochloric acid, it is an essential element of blood. The main function of this anion is to counterbalance sodium.

Chlorides are increased with acute renal failure, uremia, and urinary obstruction. Decreased serum chloride may be found in chronic renal failure, uremia, tubular acidosis, extracellular fluid excess, edema, fevers, diabetes, pneumonia and congestive heart failure.

Normal level: 97-107 mEq/L

NOTES

Chloremia, increased chloride in the blood.

Creatinine

A nitrogenous compound formed as a metabolic end product of creatine, creatinine is formed in the muscle in relatively small amounts, passes into the blood, and is excreted in the urine.

A laboratory test for creatinine level in the blood may be used as a measurement of the kidney function. Since creatinine is normally produced in fairly constant amounts due to the breakdown of phosphocreatine, and is excreted in the urine, an elevation in the creatinine level in the blood indicates a disturbance in kidney function.

The rate of urine production, muscular exercise, water intake, or protein ingestion does not affect the serum creatinine levels, which stay remarkably constant.

In the chronic hemodialysis patient, creatinine levels serve to indicate if the dialysis treatment is adequate. Dialysis time or dialyzer may be changed depending on the creatinine results.

Normal levels: 0.5-1.3 mg/dl

NOTES

Creatinine clearance test, a test of renal function based on the rate which ingested creatinine is filtered through the renal glomeruli.

Glucose

A simple sugar, also called dextrose, it is the principal monosaccharide in the human blood and body fluids.

Dialysis centers usually have protocols like weekly glucose testing on diabetic patients.

Normal level: 80-110 mg/dl

NOTES

Glucose that is not needed for energy is stored in the form of glycogen as a source of potential energy, readily available when needed. Most of the glycogen is stored in the liver and muscle cells.

HgbA1C

      Glycated hemoglobin (glycosylated hemoglobin, *hemoglobin A1c, HbA$_{1c}$, A1C*, or *Hb$_{1c}$*; sometimes also **HbA1c**) is a form of hemoglobin which is measured primarily to identify the average plasma glucose concentration over prolonged periods of time. It is formed in a non-enzymatic glycation pathway by hemoglobin's exposure to plasma glucose. Normal levels of glucose produce a normal amount of glycated hemoglobin. As the average amount of plasma glucose increases, the fraction of glycated hemoglobin increases in a predictable way. This serves as a marker for average blood glucose levels over the previous months prior to the measurement.

      The International Diabetes Federation and American College of Endocrinology recommend HbA$_{1c}$ values below 48 mmol/mol **(6.5%),** while American Diabetes Association recommends that the HbA$_{1c}$ be below 53 mmol/mol **(7.0%)** for most patients.

      Laboratory results may differ depending on the analytical technique, the age of the subject, and biological variation among individuals. Two individuals with the same average blood sugar can have A1C values that differ by as much as 3 percentage points. Results can be unreliable in many circumstances, such as after blood loss, for example, after surgery, blood transfusions, anemia, or high erythrocyte turnover; in the presence of chronic renal or liver disease; after administration of high-dose vitamin C; or erythropoetin treatment.

NOTES

Iron

Iron is the main constituent of hemoglobin and is essential in the transportation of oxygen. It is needed for tissue respiration and the development of blood cells.

Normal level: 41-132 mcg/dl

NOTES

Most iron reaches the body in food, where it occurs naturally in the form of iron compounds.

Magnesium

Excretion of excess magnesium is another normal kidney function that is lost in renal failure. Magnesium is present only in small amounts but it is important for proper cell functioning. Individuals with high levels of this electrolyte may show reduced nerve and muscle activity, which impairs respirations, produces lethargy and coma, and may result in cardiac arrest if condition is not corrected. It is important to know if the patient has been using preparations high in magnesium such as Mylanta, Maalox, milk of magnesia, or citrate of magnesium.

Normal level: 1.6-2.4 mg/dl

NOTES

It is found in the intra- and extracellular fluids and is excreted in urine and feces.

Phosphate

Phosphates are widely distributed in the body, the largest amounts being in the bones and teeth. They are continuously excreted in the urine and feces, and must be replaced in the diet.

The hemodialysis patient is given phosphate binders to help the removal of excess phosphate in the feces. High levels of phosphorus in the blood will cause calcium depletion from the bone, resulting in bone softening. Patients with this problem have a higher risk of breaking bones and require longer recovery periods.

Remember, dialysis does not correct the disordered calcium-phosphorus metabolism, and is not very effective in removing phosphate; progressive osteodystrophy is a serious problem for many chronic hemodialysis patients.

Normal level: 2.5–4.5 mg/dl

NOTES

Phosphatemia: an excess of phosphates in the blood.

Potassium

In combination with other minerals in the body, potassium forms alkaline salts that are important in the body processes and play an essential part in the maintenance of the acid-base and water balance in the body.
All body cells, especially muscle tissue, require a high content of potassium. A proper balance between sodium, calcium, and potassium in the blood plasma is necessary for proper cardiac functioning.
In the dialysis population, hyperkalemia is a common problem and usually is diet-related. Many patients have to dialyze on an emergency basis for this reason, but is not the only reason for heperkalemia. Severe tissue or cell damage and destruction will also cause the potassium level of the blood to rise since potassium is found in large amounts in the intracellular fluid. *
Hypokalemia is also a problem due to problem due to prolonged vomiting and diarrhea.
Dialysate potassium concentration should be adjusted depending on the patient's serum potassium level.

Normal level: 3.5-5.0 mEq/L

* Kayexalate is a potassium-removing resin used in the treatment of hyperkalemia when dialysis is contradicted or unavailable. It can be given orally or by enema.

Sodium

Sodium is the major extracellular cation. It plays a dominant role in controlling acid-base equilibrium and the balance of water between blood and body tissue cells. Hemodialysis patients may have a low sodium level due to fluid overload (dilution hyponatremia).

Low levels of this electrolyte can cause muscle cramping and high levels can cause excessive thirst.

Normal level: 135-145 mEq/L

NOTES

Sodium constitutes 90 to 95% of all cations in the blood plasma and interstitial fluid.

Uric Acid

This is the end product of purine (*a colorless crystalline compound*) metabolism in the body; the waste product is excreted in the urine. In gout, there is an excess of uric acid in the blood. The salt of uric acid forms insoluble stones in the urinary tract, or may crystallize and form deposits in the joints and tissues.

Normal level: **6.9-7.5 mg/100 ml**

NOTES

Uric: pertaining to the urine.

Normal Chemistries*

Albumin		3.6-5.0 g/dl
Bicarbonate	HCO3	24-31 mEq/L
Blood urea nitrogen	BUN	6-25 mg/dl
Calcium	Ca++	8.5-10.5 mg/dl
Chloride	Cl-	97-107 mEq/L
Creatinine		0.5-1.3 mg/dl
Glucose		80-110 mg/dl
Iron	Fe++	41-132 mg/dl
Magnesium	Mg++	1.6-2.4 mg/dl
Phosphorus	PO4	2.5-4.5 mg/dl
Potassium	K+	3.5-5.0 mEq/l
Serum glutamic oxalacetic transaminase	SGOT	5-33 IU/L
Serum glutamic pyruvic transaminase	SGPT	1-33 IU/L
Sodium	Na+	135-145 mEq/L
Total Protein	Pr-	5.5-8.0 g/dl
Uric acid		6.9-7.5 mg/100 ml

	Male	Female
WBC	4.8 – 10.8	4.8 – 10.8
RBC	4.7 – 6.1	4.2 – 5.4
HGB	14.0 –18.0	12.0 – 16.0
HCT	42 - 52	37 – 47

Laboratory values may differ among institutions.

The only thing in life achieved without effort is failure.

- Unknown

Chapter 7

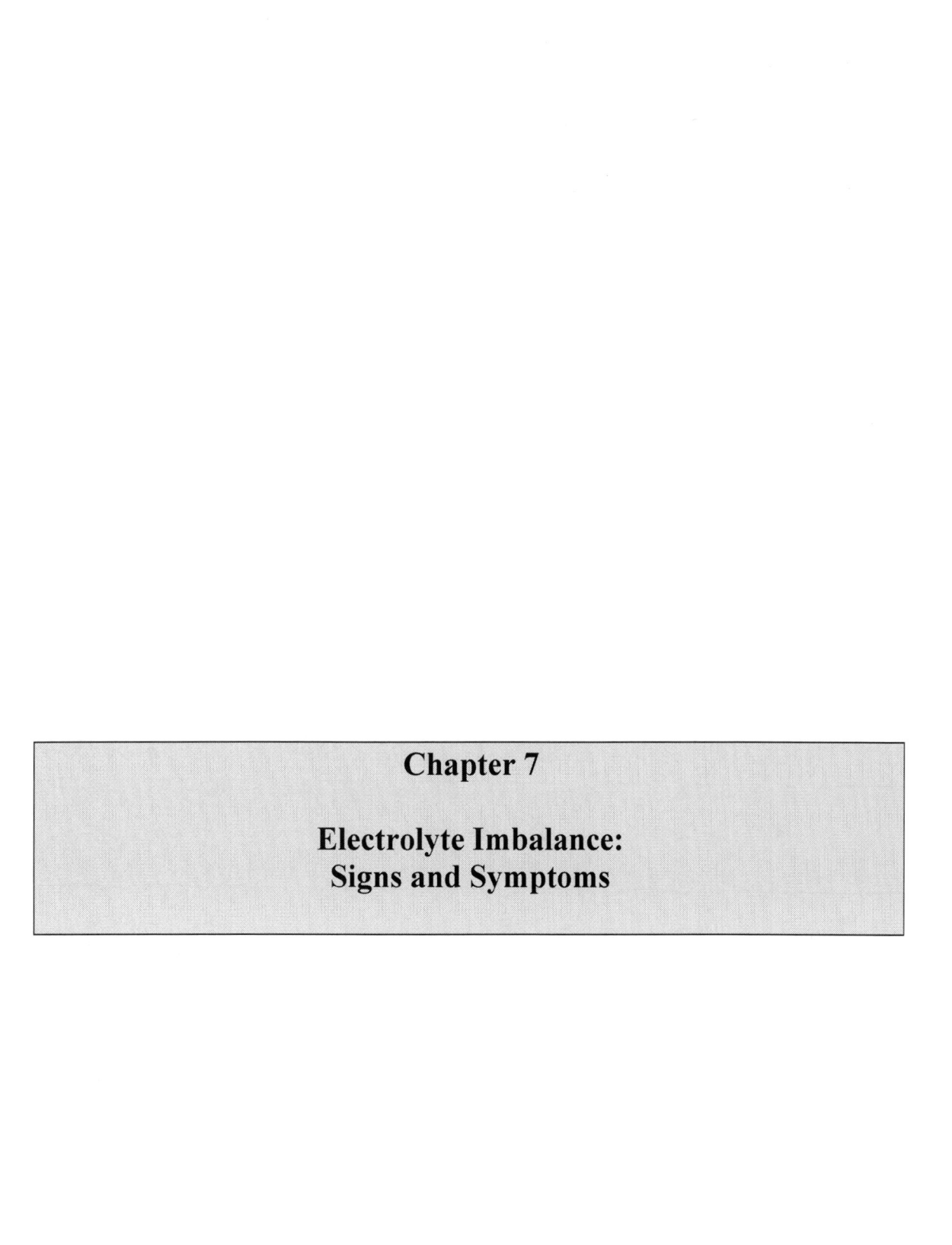

Electrolyte Imbalance: Signs and Symptoms

Calcium Deficit   **Hypocalcemia**

    a. Abdominal cramps
    b. Harsh, high-pitched, respiratory sounds (laryngeal stridor)
    c. Hyperactive reflexes
    d. Numbness
    e. Spasms of feet and wrist (carpopedal spasms)
    f. Tetany
    g. Tingling around mouth
    h. Tingling of the ends of the fingers

NOTES

Hypocalcemia is best corrected with both oral calcium and oral calcitriol.

| **Calcium Excess** | **Hypercalcemia** |

a. Anorexia
b. Azotemia
c. Cardiac irregularities
d. Deep-bone pain
e. Flank pain
f. Formation of cavities in the bone
g. Kidney stones
h. Lethargy
i. Muscle hypotonicity
j. Nausea, vomiting
k. Weight loss

NOTES

Hypercalcemia is associated with hyperparathyroidism.
A common but infrequently described problem that may cause acute hypercalcemia in the previously stable uremic patient is bed rest. When a normal patient goes to bed, bone formation decreases rapidly and bone re-absorption slows down less quickly.

Magnesium Deficit — **Hypomagnesemia**

a. Convulsions
b. Disorientation
c. Hyperactive deep reflexes
d. Tremor

NOTES

Manifested chiefly by neuromuscular hyperirritability.

Potassium Deficit	**Hypokalemia**

a. Cardiac irregularities
b. Diminished to absent reflexes
c. Faint heart sounds
d. Falling blood pressure
e. Fatigability
f. Generalized weakness
g. Increased sensitivity to digitalis
h. Shallow respirations
i. Shortness of breath
j. Vomiting
k. Weak pulse

NOTES

The EKG abnormalities presented are depression of the T wave and elevation of the U wave. Susceptibility to digitalis toxicity is increased when a patient has hypokalemia.

| **Potassium Excess** | **Hyperkalemia** |

a. Cardiac irregularities
b. Diarrhea
c. Dizziness
d. Intestinal colic
e. Irritability
f. Muscle cramps
g. Muscle pain
h. Nausea
i. Weakness

NOTES

Potassium levels grater than 7 mEq/L can produce EKG abnormalities evident first as peaked T waves and depressed P waves, widened QRS waves, and eventual asystole.

| **Sodium Deficit** | **Hyponatremia** |

- a. Apprehension
- b. Cramps
- c. Convulsions
- d. Fatigue
- e. Muscular weakness

NOTES

When the cause of hyponatremia is salt wasting there is an accompanying loss of body fluids. Treatment is based on correction of the underlying cause.

Sodium Excess | **Hypernatremia**

a. Dry skin
b. Dry, sticky, mucous membrane
c. Elevated body temperature
d. Flushed skin
e. Rough, dry tongue
f. Thirst

NOTES

Indicative of water loss exceeding the sodium loss.

Chapter 8

Potential Problems
In Hemodialysis

TROUBLESHOOTING
Air Embolus

The alarm in a dialysis machine goes off, you find the alarming machine and see that the air detector light is on. You look at the bloodlines and see air in the venous line.

Your *first* intervention will be:

Your reasoning for your intervention:

Air Embolus

Causes

- a. Air detector left off or not functioning
- b. Air leak in blood tubing or connections before the blood pump
- c. Careless fluid administration

Signs and Symptoms

- a. Patient complaints of tightness in chest or dyspnea
- b. Patient becomes cyanotic
- c. Foam detected in blood tubing

Medical and Nursing Interventions

- b. Clamp blood line
- b. Stop blood pump
- c. Lower patient's head and patient to left side
- d. Notify physician immediately
- e. If possible, save extracorporeal blood by recirculating blood or blood bagging
- f. Keep the patient on left side and in Trendelenburg until air embolus is ruled out

Expected Outcomes

- a. Patient verbalizes no symptoms related to this problem
- b. No evidence of cough or cyanosis
- c. No cardiac arrest

Reminder

The use of some single needle devices with a high blood flow may cause foam in the extracorporeal system.

TROUBLESHOOTING
Angina

You are making rounds in the dialysis center. You see a patient laying in the chair feeling anxious. You check the blood pressure and the patient is hypotensive. When you ask the patient how she is feeling she verbalizes having chest pain.

Your *first* intervention will be:

Your reasoning for your intervention:

Angina

Causes

    a.   Anxiety
    b.   Hypotension
    c.   Increasing blood flow too rapidly in patients with known cardiac disease

Signs and Symptoms

    a.   Patient verbalizes chest pain or burning sensation

Medical and Nursing Interventions

    a.   Start I.V. fluid administration, discontinue ultrafiltration
    b.   Provide sedatives or antianginal medication as indicated
    c.   To prevent angina, increase blood flow slowly at beginning of dialysis

Expected Outcomes

    a.   Patient verbalizes no chest pain

Reminder

    Sedatives or antianginal medications may cause hypotension; check BP every 15 minutes and PRN until stable.

TROUBLESHOOTING
Arm Pain

You are talking to a fellow worker in the middle of the dialysis center when a patient calls your name. You respond to his call and ask what is the problem. The patient complaints of pain at the needle sites.

Your intervention will be:

Your reasoning for your intervention:

Arm Pain

Causes

    a.   Immobility for a prolonged time
    b.   Needle position
    c.   Trauma at needle site

Signs and Symptoms

    a.   Complaints of pain, numbness, or throbbing in arm

Medical and Nursing Interventions

    a.   Avoid traumatic needle insertion
    b.   In the event of arm pain:
- readjust the needle
- readjust arm position
- apply heating pad or warm towel (Use caution with diabetic patients)
- medicate per order
- consider needle replacement

Expected Outcomes

    a.   Patient verbalizes minimal or no pain

Reminder

Consider using armboard to secure the fistula needles better.

TROUBLESHOOTING
Bleeding AV Access

You are going to cannulate the arm on Mr. Jones and you read the last treatment sheet in which states the patient bled for over 30 minutes on his last dialysis treatment.

You intervention will be:

Your reasoning for your intervention:

Bleeding AV Access

Causes

    a. Over-heparinization
    b. Prolonged clotting time
    c. Too little pressure at puncture site
    d. Trauma
    e. Weakening in the wall (aneurysm)

Signs and Symptoms

    a. Bleeding at puncture site
    b. Formation of hematoma at puncture site

Medical and Nursing Interventions

    a. Avoid trauma and tissue damage by smooth needle insertion
    b. Rotate needle sites and use side vessels
    c. In the event of bleeding
- adjust applied pressure
- apply Gelfoam or topical thrombin
- consider giving IV Protamine
- perform clotting times next dialysis and adjust heparin as indicated

Expected Outcomes

    No bleeding after ten minutes

Reminder

    Rebound may occur when Protamine is used and bleeding may continue.

TROUBLESHOOTING
Blood Loss

Your are making rounds in the dialysis center on the second shift of patients. While you are taking the blood pressure on a patient the alarm goes off on the next station. You look and see that is the Arterial Monitor alarm.

The patient's arms are covered with a blanket so you, at the first glance, can't see the needles in the access arm. You look down and see blood on the floor.

Your *first* intervention will be:

Your reasoning for your intervention:

Blood Loss

Causes

    a. Blood line separation
    b. Dialyzer leak or rupture
    c. AV fistula needle dislodgment

Sign and Symptoms

    a. Activated blood detector alarm
    b. Leaking at needle sites
    c. Air in blood lines past the point of separation

Medical and Nursing Interventions

    a. If any question of leak, check dialysate with Hemastix
    b. In the event of a *small* hollow-fiber leak
- reduce negative pressure for 15-20 minutes to allow leaking fibers to clot
- recheck with Hemastix; if negative, gradually increase negative pressure and again check with Hemastix
- If unable to seal leak, replace hollow fiber

    c. In the event of a parallel plate leak
- reduce negative pressure
- return the blood, maintaining some positive pressure in the blood compartment to avoid contamination of the blood by dialysate
- replace the parallel plate

    d. Evaluate blood loss, patient's hematocrit, and need for blood transfusion

Expected Outcomes

    Resolution of blood loss

Reminder

    In older machines, if using dry ultrafiltration, the blood detector may be bypassed and blood leak may not be detected. Check ultrafiltrate frequently with Hemastix. In the event of a blood leak, save the lot number of the dialyzer for future reference as it may be a defective lot. Maintain a positive venous pressure, otherwise, dialysate can go into the blood compartment of the dialyzer.

TROUBLESHOOTING
Blood Transfusion Reaction

You are replacing the bicarbonate container on a dialysis machine because is running low. The patient on this machine is getting a blood transfusion. The patient complaints to you about having chills and nausea, and feeling like she will vomit any time.

Your intervention will be:

Your reasoning for your intervention:

Blood Transfusion Reaction

Causes

    a.   Anaphylactic or allergic reaction
    b.   Circulatory overload
    c.   Hemolytic reaction
    e.   Pyrogenic or bacterial reaction

Signs and Symptoms

    a.   Hemolytic reaction (occurs within 15 min. of starting transfusion)
- heat along vein, flushed face, pain in chest, lumbar region and abdomen, nausea, vomiting, headache, shock, fever, chills

    b.   Circulatory overload (occurs during transfusion)
- dyspnea, rales, rhonchi, frothy sputum, cyanosis, pulmonary edema, lung hemorrhage

    c.   Pyrogenic or bacterial reaction (occurs near end of or after transfusion)
- headache, nausea, vomiting, pain in lumbar region or muscle pain, fever, chills

    d.   Anaphylactic or allergic reaction (occurs early in the transfusion or at any time during subsequent transfusions)
- Wheals, hives, urticaria, erythema, chills, asthmatic-type wheezing, laryngeal edema, and respiratory distress

Medical and Nursing Interventions

    a.   Stop blood immediately
    b.   Keep vein open
    c.   Change IV tubing immediately
    d.   Notify physician
    e.   Notify laboratory
    f.   Monitor vital signs Q5 min. and as needed
    g.   Send blood bag, blood tubing, and transfusion report to laboratory
    h.   Send first urine passed after reaction to lab for analysis
    i.   Record the events and interventions taken in the nurses' notes

Expected Outcomes

    a.   Absence of or decrease in the signs and symptoms
    b.   Patient's vital signs stable

TROUBLESHOOTING
Blood Vessel Spasm

You are sitting in the nursing station charting on your last patient's take-off and a patient calls your name. You go to him and complaints of pain along the vein where the fistula needles are placed.

Your intervention will be:

Your reasoning for your intervention:

Blood Vessel Spasm

Causes

    Irritation of blood vessel by cold normal saline or albumin

Signs and Symptoms

    a.   Complaints of pain or cold along vessel path
    b.   Venous resistance higher than usual for patient

Medical and Nursing Intervention

    a.   Avoid giving cold normal saline or albumin
    b.   Apply heating pad or warm towel to affected area. (**WARNING:** Temperature can be to hot for some patients, especially for diabetic patients, causing damage to the tissue)

Expected Outcomes

    No evidence of vessel spasm.

TROUBLESHOOTING
Bone Disease

You are reviewing the monthly laboratory results and find that the Phosphorus levels are 9.5 mg/dL. The patient had also a bone fracture of the right lower extremity two weeks ago.

Your intervention will be:

Your reasoning for your intervention:

Bone Disease

Causes

    a. Calcium-phosphate imbalance
    b. Decreased calcium intake, calcium malabsorption
    c. Hyperphosphatemia
    d. Inefficient dialysis
    e. Low calcium concentration in the dialysate

Signs and Symptoms

    a. Evidence of bone degeneration per x-ray
    b. Incidence of pathological fractures
    c. Elevated phosphate level (serum)

Medical and Nursing Interventions

    a. Review medication dosage and importance
    b. Review status of disease process and safety precautions to be taken
    c. Request dietary consult regarding calcium/phosphorus intake
    d. Review lab values and check for high serum phosphate and calcium
    e. Increase phosphate binders
    f. Increase calcium in dialysate

Expected Outcomes

    a. No evidence of bone degeneration per x-ray
    b. Patient verbalizes correct medication and diet and their importance

TROUBLESHOOTING
Cardiac Dysrhythmias

You are making your hourly rounds in the unit, checking the vitals and the machines. A patient complaints to you of chest pain. You take the pulse and it is irregular.

Your intervention will be:

Your reasoning for your intervention:

Cardiac Dysrhythmias

Causes

- a. Congestive heart failure
- b. Digoxin toxicity
- c. Electrolyte imbalance (i.e., rapid shift in serum potassium or sodium)
- d. Emotions
- e. Hyperkalemia
- f. Hypotension
- g. Volume excess

Signs and Symptoms

- a. Complaints of chest pain or fluttering sensation in chest
- b. Dysrhytmias on cardiac monitor
- c. Irregular heartbeat

Medical and Nursing Interventions

a. Check apical pulse
b. In the event of dysrhytmias
- Draw stat potassium
- Adjust potassium content of dialysate to avoid rapid shift
- Run rhythm shift
- Report to physician
- Medicate with antidysrhytmic drug(s) per order
- Request dietary consult

TROUBLESHOOTING
Clotting in Dialyzer

A dialysis machine alarms, you respond quickly and find that the alarm indicates a high venous resistance. You also note that clots are forming in the venous chamber.

Your intervention will be:

Your reasoning for your intervention:

Clotting in Dialyzer

Causes

    a.   Blood not circulating through the extracorporeal system for a time (i.e., when replacing a fistula needle, mechanical failure, etc.)
    b.   Improper heparinization
    c.   Improper prime

Signs and Symptoms

    a.   Increased venous resistance (if clotting occurs below the venous chamber)
    b.   Fibers darkening in the dialyzer

Medical and Nursing Interventions

    a.   Administer more heparin
    b.   Performed activated clotting time (ACT) every half-to one hour as indicated
    c.   If mechanical failure occurs, hand crank blood pump
    d.   Check heparin pump at least every half-hour for proper infusion
    e.   Make sure dialyzer is primed properly

Expected Outcomes

    a.   No loss of dialyzer
    b.   No dialyzer surface loss
    c.   No blood loss

Reminder

    If blood recirculation is needed, use a connector to connect the venous and arterial bloodlines.

TROUBLESHOOTING
Cramps

A patient screams loudly, jumps out of the recliner complaining of severe muscle cramps in his legs.

Your *first* intervention will be:

Your reasoning for your intervention:

Cramps

Causes

    a. Fluid depletion
    b. Ischemia
    c. Sodium shift

Signs and Symptoms

    a. Complaints of tingling sensation
    b. Cramps

Medical and Nursing Interventions

    a. Give high sodium bath or sodium modeling (if possible)
    b. Check blood pressure every ½ hour and PRN
    c. Request dietary consult regarding sodium intake
    d. In the event of cramps
- apply local heat
- massage area and apply local pressure
- give normal saline IV (0.9%)
- decrease blood flow
- give Mannitol, glucose 50%, or concentrated saline IV push if indicated
- give quinine sulfate prior to dialysis

Expected Outcomes

Absent or minimal cramps

Reminder

Glucose may not be indicated in diabetic patients. Consult the physician prior to giving medications. Follow unit's protocol.

TROUBLESHOOTING
Dyspnea

You are passing the charts for the third shift of patients, while placing the chart behind a machine you notice a patient having difficulty breathing and to you, he looks cyanotic.

Your *first* intervention will be:

Your reasoning for your intervention:

Dyspnea

Causes

    a. Air embolus
    b. Dialyzer contents returned too rapidly at the end of dialysis
    c. Fluid excess

Signs and Symptoms

    a. Difficult breathing or tightness in chest
    b. Cyanosis
    c. Rapid, labored respiration

Medical and Nursing Interventions

    a. Observe for air in the extracorporeal system
    b. Ultrafiltrate for excess fluid
    c. Return dialyzer contents slowly, especially in patients with known cardiac disease
    d. Oxygen may be used to lessen the symptoms

Expected Outcomes

    Respiratory distress diminished or absent.

TROUBLESHOOTING
Eye Changes

You have a patient that you have been dialyzing for five years. She has Diabetes Type II and history of Hypertension. The patient is now complaining to you that she is having problems reading the newspaper.

Your intervention will be:

Your reasoning for your intervention:

Eye Changes

Causes

    a. Diabetes
    b. Hemodialysis

Signs and Symptoms

    a. Decreased visual acuity
    b. Retinal hemorrhages noted on examination

Medical and Nursing Interventions

    a. Reduce heparin infusion during dialysis treatment
    b. Assess and give amount of assistance patient needs for the activities of daily living
    c. Ensure comfort and safety
    d. Patients may undergo various types of treatment to improve or correct eye problems (i.e., laser treatments, surgery)

Expected Outcomes

    a. Patient verbalizes comfort and security with assistance provided
    b. Stabilization of eye changes
    c. Improvement of eyesight

TROUBLESHOOTING
Fever/Chills

The automatic blood pressure machine indicates that the blood pressure is dropping on your patient, he is also having chills. The patient has been dialyzing for 45 minutes.

Your intervention will be:

Your reasoning for your intervention:

Fever /Chills

Causes

- a. Pyrogen reaction – diffusion of bacterial toxin across membrane into blood (usually occurs within the first hour of dialysis)
- b. Transfusion reaction

Signs and Symptoms

- a. Headache, itching, chest pain
- b. Fever, chills, hypotension, hives, shortness of breath

Medical and Nursing Intervention

- a. Send blood cultures, inflow-outflow dialysate cultures, and water source culture to the laboratory
- b. Monitor temperature and blood pressure
- c. Give antipyretic drugs as indicated
- d. Discontinue dialysis if symptoms do not subside
- e. If blood transfusion reaction, discontinue transfusion (See blood transfusion reaction)

Expected Outcomes

Patient verbalizes no complaints of signs and symptoms.

TROUBLESHOOTING
Headache

You are taking care of four patients, this is your first shift in the early morning and a patient calls you to tell you that she has a "terrible" headache.

Your intervention will be:

Your reasoning for your intervention:

Headache

Causes

    a. Disequilibrium
    b. Emotional problems
    c. Hypertension
    d. Physical problem, non-dialysis related

Signs and Symptoms

    Headache, nausea

Medical and Nursing Interventions

    a. Slowly increase blood flow
    b. Slowly increase ultrafiltration
    c. Medicate per order
    d. Give Mannitol in normal saline, slow IV drip during dialysis
    e. Give antihypertensive drug therapy
    f. Provide shorter and more frequent treatments

Expected Outcomes

    Patient verbalizes absence of or minimal headache.

TROUBLESHOOTING
Hemolysis

A female patient on machine number 24 calls your name, as you walk towards the station you can hear the patient complaining of chest pain. You look at the extracorporeal system and you notice that the blood in the venous line has a cherry-colored look to it.

Your *first* intervention will be:

Your reasoning for your intervention:

Hemolysis

Causes

- a. Cleaning agent within dialysate system
- b. Improper dialysate preparation due to mechanical failure or human error
- c. Limits not set on conductivity meter (old machines)
- d. Over-occluded blood pump
- e. Over-heated dialysate

Signs and Symptoms

- a. Chest pain, dyspnea, hypotension, and possible shock
- b. Blood is cherry-colored and is translucent when put in light, or serum is pink to red when blood is centrifuged

Medical and Nursing Interventions

- a. Have a systematic procedure for setting up and checking equipment to avoid errors
- b. If hemolysis occurs when *initiating* dialysis, discard blood in dialyzer and correct dialysate before restarting; evaluate need for transfusions
- c. If hemolysis occurs during treatment, stop dialysate flow and/or treatment until dialysate concentration can be corrected; check patient's hematocrit and transfuse as necessary
- d. In the event of hemolysis, do stat serum potassium level
- e. Maintain blood pressure with normal saline or albumin
- f. Give oxygen PRN

Expected Outcomes

- a. Patient verbalizes no complaints of signs and symptoms
- b. Blood show no signs of hemolysis

Reminder

Before starting treatment, always check dialysate for the presence of bleach or formalin and take a conductivity reading. Make sure temperature is within normal limits.

TROUBLESHOOTING
Hypertension

You are making blood pressure rounds in your second shift of patients. As you take the blood pressure manually, the patient complaints to you of a severe headache. His blood pressure is 196/102. You take it again and it is about the same.

Your intervention will be:

Your reasoning for your intervention:

Hypertension

Causes

    a. Anxiety
    b. Disequilibrium syndrome
    c. Volume overload due to excess sodium and fluid intake

Signs and Symptoms

    a. Blood pressure elevated above patient's norm
    b. Headache, nausea, or vomiting
    c. Weight gain above the patient's norm

Medical and Nursing Interventions

    a. If disequilibrium syndrome is the cause, slow or discontinue dialysis
    b. Provide vigorous ultrafiltration
    c. Do dry ultrafiltration (Isolated UF)
    d. Give antihypertensive drug therapy
    e. Sedate patient, if related to anxiety

Expected Outcomes

    a. Blood pressure returns to patient's norm
    b. Weight decreased to patient's estimated dry weight

TROUBLESHOOTING
Hypotension

You are passing the lab results to the charts located with the patients as they are dialyzing. You see an older male patient with his eyes close, you wonder if he is OK or just at sleep. You touch his shoulder and the patient does not respond.

Your *first* intervention will be:

Your reasoning for your intervention:

Hypotension

Causes

    a. Congestive heart failure
    b. Eating
    c. Fluid depletion
    d. Fluid depletion secondary to dialyzer fill
    e. Presence of two access sites (i.e., two functional fistulas)
    f. Vascular system status

Signs and Symptoms

    a. Nausea and vomiting
    b. Blurred vision
    c. Drop in patient's normal blood pressure
    d. Loss of consciousness
    e. Seizure

Medical and Nursing Interventions

    a. Check patient's blood pressure every half-hour and more often if needed
    b. Check patient's weight every two hours (if possible)
    c. Fill dialyzer slowly
    d. Provide small meals or no meals during dialysis
    e. Give normal saline or albumin prime
    f. Decrease or eliminate ultrafiltration; dry ultrafiltration may be tolerated better for high removal of fluid in a short time
    g. Treat hypotension with normal saline or albumin until blood pressure is stable at patient's norm
    h. Place patient in the Trendelenburg position

Expected Outcomes

    a. Patient remains mormotensive
    b. Weight does not drop below patient's dry weight

TROUBLESHOOTING
Infection

You are about to cannulate a patient so you can start the hemodialysis treatment on her as soon as possible because you are running late. As you clean the arm where the graft is located you see drainage from an exit site. You know a CBC was done two days back as part of the monthly blood work. You find the lab report on her chart and see that her WBC count is 18,000.

Your intervention will be:

Your reasoning for your intervention:

Infection

Causes

    a. Decreased resistance
    b. Inadequate septic solution
    c. Poor care of access
    d. Poor needle technique

Signs and Symptoms

    a. Redness or swelling at exit site
    b. Elevated WBC count
    c. Local or generalized elevation of temperature
    d. Drainage at exit site

Medical and Nursing Interventions

    a. In the event of infection
- obtain blood cultures
- obtain complete blood count (CBC)
- antibiotic therapy may be indicated

    b. Review needle technique
    c. Provide care of puncture sites post-dialysis
    d. Use proper septic solution
    e. Review procedures for care of dialysis catheters
    f. Explain to patient about her/his decreased resistance and precautions to be taken

Expected Outcomes

    No signs and symptoms of local infection

TROUBLESHOOTING
Nausea and Vomiting

This may not be your day because as you get close to a patient having dialysis, he vomits in a projectile manner, which hits your lab coat.

Your first intervention will be:

Your reason for your intervention:

Nausea and Vomiting

Causes

    a. Gastrointestinal disturbances
    b. Hypotension
    c. Physical or emotional disequilibrium

Signs and Symptoms

    Nausea, vomiting

Medical and Nursing Interventions

    a. Decrease blood flow rate (QB)
    b. Remove ultrafiltration (UF)
    c. Medicate patient if ordered
    d. If hypotensive, give IV fluids
    e. To *prevent* nausea and vomiting
- Prevent hypotension
- Provide small meals or no meals during dialysis
- Request dietary consult

Expected Outcomes

    a. Patient verbalizes no complaints of nausea
    b. No evidence of vomiting

Reminder

    Vomiting may cause potassium deficit; check patient's K level; be alert to signs and symptoms of hypokalemia

TROUBLESHOOTING
Neuropathy

As you are taking the patient's weight he complaints to you of having weakness in his legs. His serum potassium is in the normal limits.

Your intervention will be:

Your reasoning for your intervention:

Neuropathy

Causes

    a.   Central nervous system disturbances
    b.   Inadequate dialysis

Signs and Symptoms

    a.   Burning, pain, or weakness in extremities
    b.   Decreased nerve conduction velocity per Nerve Conduction Study (NCS)
    c.   May complaint of weakness in legs

Medical and Nursing Interventions

    a.   Ensure maximum blood flow rate during hemodialysis
    b.   Increase dialysis time
    c.   Explain disease process and safety precautions to be taken
    d.   Re-evaluate type and size of dialyzer being used

Expected Outcomes

    a.   Patient is free of burning, pain, or weakness in extremities
    b.   NCS shows no decrease in nerve conduction velocity

TROUBLESHOOTING
Power Failure

It is Monday morning and the first shift of patients are on the machines having dialysis. All 26 stations are full today. It has been raining all night, a big storm was coming from the North-West. Suddenly, the lights go out and all the dialysis machines are alarming. The dialysis center lost the power and they don't have an emergency generator.

Your intervention will be:

Your reasoning for your intervention:

Power Failure

Causes

- a. Disaster resulting in electrical cutoff
- b. Overloading of electrical system

Signs and Symptoms

- a. Shut down of all electrical equipment
- b. Equipment alarms activated

Medical and Nursing Interventions

- a. Maintain blood flow with hand crank
- b. Identify and correct overloaded circuit
- c. Discontinue dialysis if unable to regain power for extended period of time

Expected Outcomes

- a. No evidence of electrical overload
- b. Prevention of blood clotting in extracorporeal system

Reminder

Some patients may need to be transfer to another facility for the dialysis treatments. Water and dialysate on the floor or around the working area can contribute to power failure; keep area dry

TROUBLESHOOTING
Pruritus

Your dialysis center, to save money, purchased a cheaper dialyzer with a cellulose membrane. Twenty-five minutes after you connected your third patient to the dialysis machine, he complaints of sever itching.

Your intervention will be:

Your reasoning for your intervention:

Pruritus

Causes

    a.   Drug or blood transfusion reaction
    b.   Inadequate dialysis time
    c.   Reaction to dialyzer
    d.   Uremia

Signs and Symptoms

    Itching or burning sensation

Medical and Nursing Interventions

    a.   Increase dialysis time
    b.   Discontinue blood transfusion or drug
    c.   Discontinue the particular dialyzer and use a more biocompatible type
    d.   Medicate with antipruritic drugs as indicated

Expected Outcomes

    Patient verbalizes minimal or no itching

TROUBLESHOOTING
Seizures

A female patient, with the history of seizures, tells you that she is starting to have muscle twitching.

Your first intervention will be:

Your reasoning for your intervention:

Seizures

Causes

    a.   Disequilibrium
    b.   Epilepsy
    c.   Hypotension
    d.   Mechanical dysfunction

Signs and Symptoms

    a.   Patient complaints of aura or muscle twitching
    b.   Petit mal seizures
    c.   Grand mal seizures

Medical and Nursing Interventions

    a.   Prevent hypotension
    b.   Check medication orders and schedule
    c.   In the event of a seizure
- Check airway; insert one if indicated
- Give normal saline
- Prevent injury to the patient
- Decrease blood flow
- Check blood pressure every 15 minutes and PRN
- Medicate patient as ordered
- Note time and length of seizure
- Note body movements involved
- Discontinue dialysis

Expected Outcomes

    Seizures absent or controlled

Reminder

    Keep tongue depressor readily available at all times; tape to bedside table, bed wall, or machine

*Success seems largely a matter of hanging on
after others have let go.*

- William Feather

Chapter 9

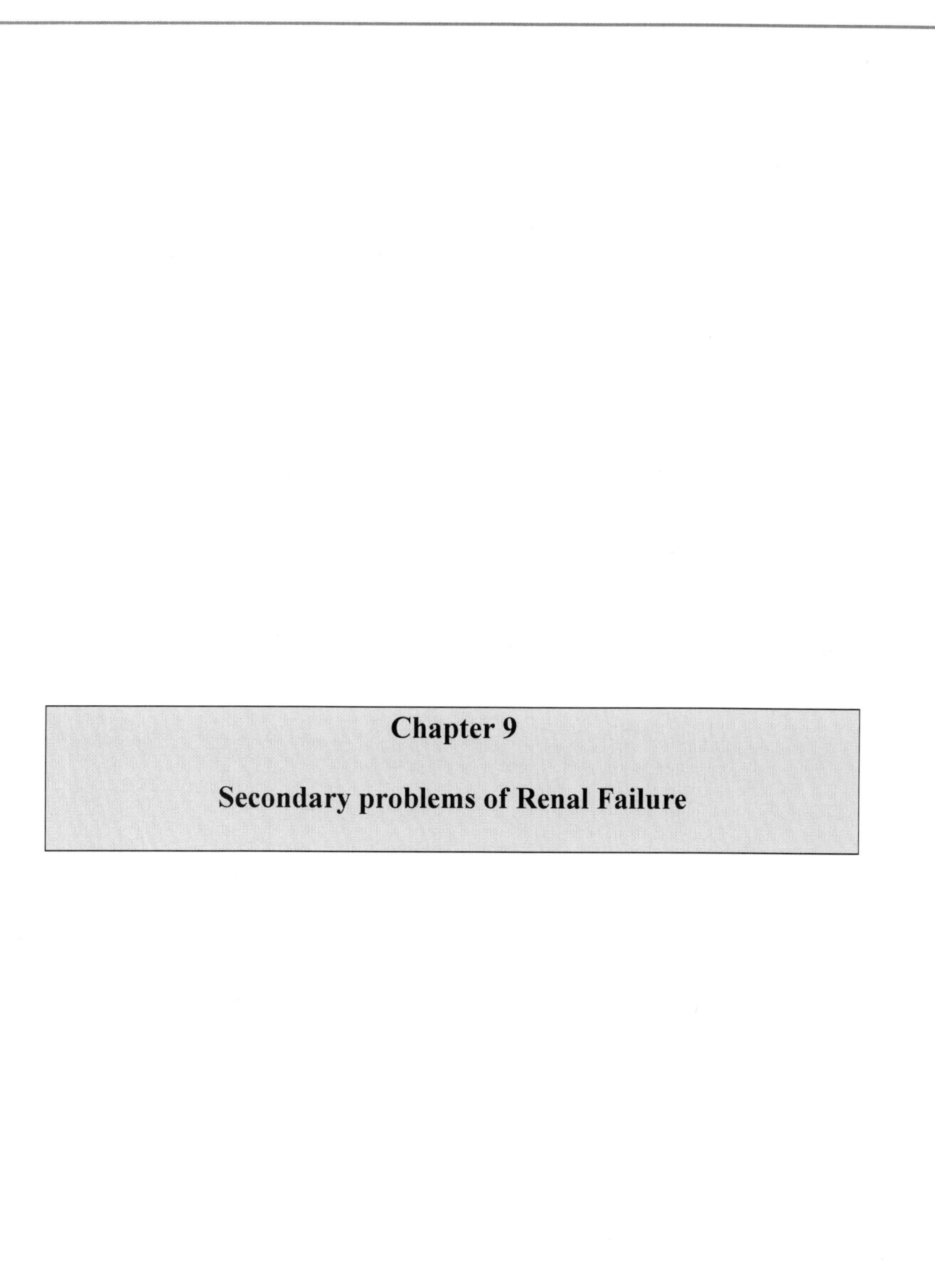

Secondary problems of Renal Failure

Cardiovascular

- **a.** Congestive heart failure
- **b.** Hypertension
- **c.** Uremic lung
- **d.** Pericarditis
- **e.** Myocardiopathy

NOTES

Pertaining to the heart and blood vessels.

Dermatological

- **a.** Pigmentation
- **b.** Pruritus
- **c.** Pallor
- **d.** Ecchymosis
- **e.** Calcium deposition
- **f.** Excoriations
- **g.** Uremic frost

NOTES

Affecting the skin.

Endocrine

- **a.** Infertility
- **b.** Sexual dysfunction
- **c.** Amenorrhea
- **d.** Hyperparathyroidism
- **e.** Thyroid abnormalities

NOTES

Pertaining to internal secretions; hormonal.

Gastrointestinal

a. Nausea
b. Vomiting
c. Anorexia
d. Peptic ulcer
e. GI bleeding
f. Gastroenteritis

NOTES

Pertaining to the stomach and intestines.

Hemotologic

a. Internal bleeding
b. Anemia

NOTES

Related to blood.

Metabolic

a. Gout
b. Hyperlipidemia
c. Malnutrition
d. Carbohydrate intolerance

NOTES

Related to processes concerned with the disposition of the nutrients absorbed into the blood following digestion.

Neurological

- **a.** Fatigue
- **b.** Headache
- **c.** Lethargy
- **d.** Muscular irritability
- **e.** Seizures
- **f.** Sleep disturbances
- **g.** Coma

NOTES

Related to the nervous system.

Ocular

a. Hypertensive retinopathy
b. Red eye syndrome
c. Band keratopathy

NOTES

Pertaining to the eye.

Peripheral Neuropathy

a. Motor weakness
b. Paresthesias
c. Restless leg syndrome
d. Paralysis

NOTES

A general term denoting functional disturbances and pathologic changes in the peripheral nervous system.

Psychological

a. Denial
b. Anxiety
c. Depression
d. Psychosis

NOTES

Related to the mind and mental processes, especially in relation to human and animal behavior.

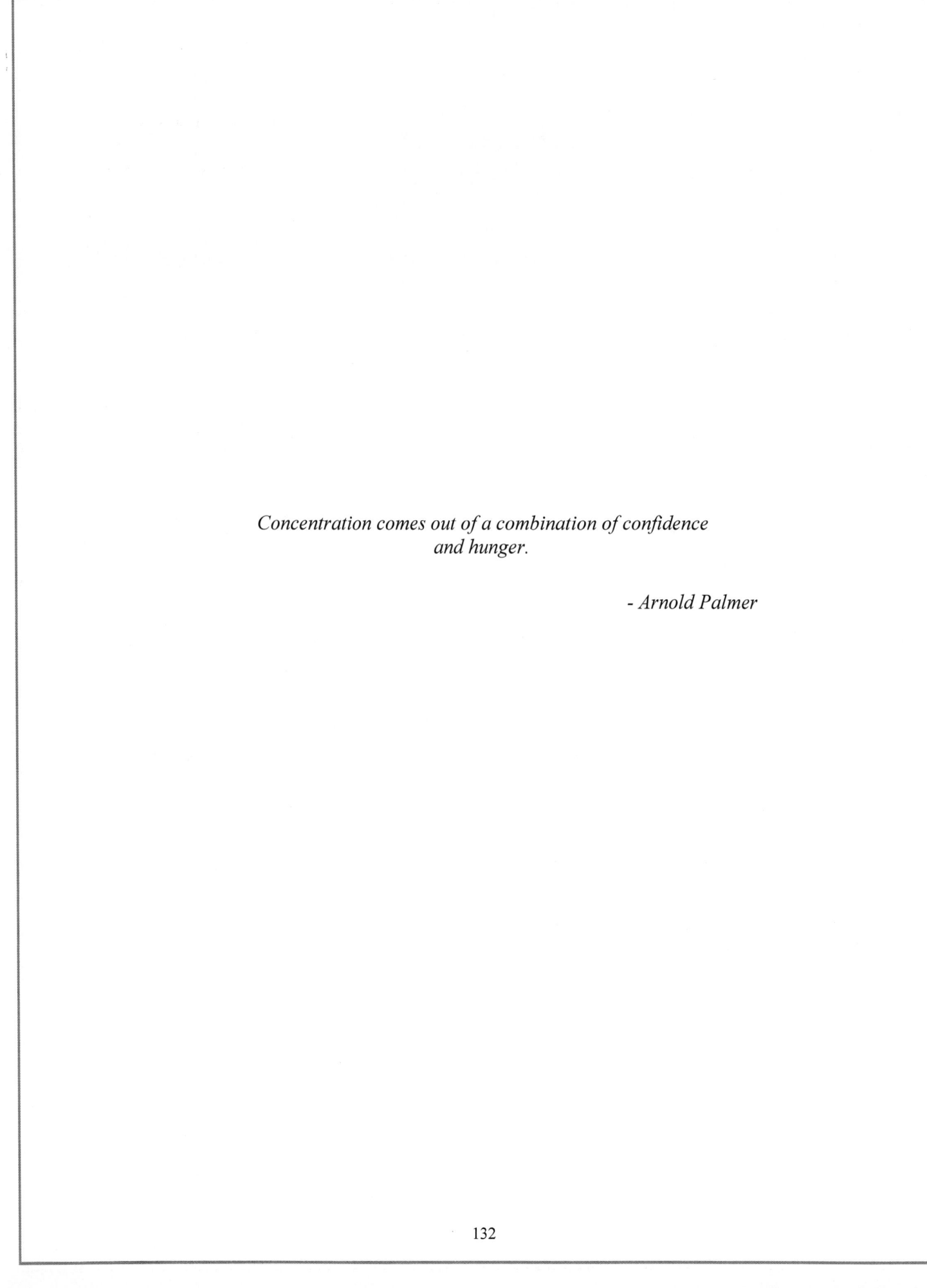

*Concentration comes out of a combination of confidence
and hunger.*

- Arnold Palmer

Chapter 10

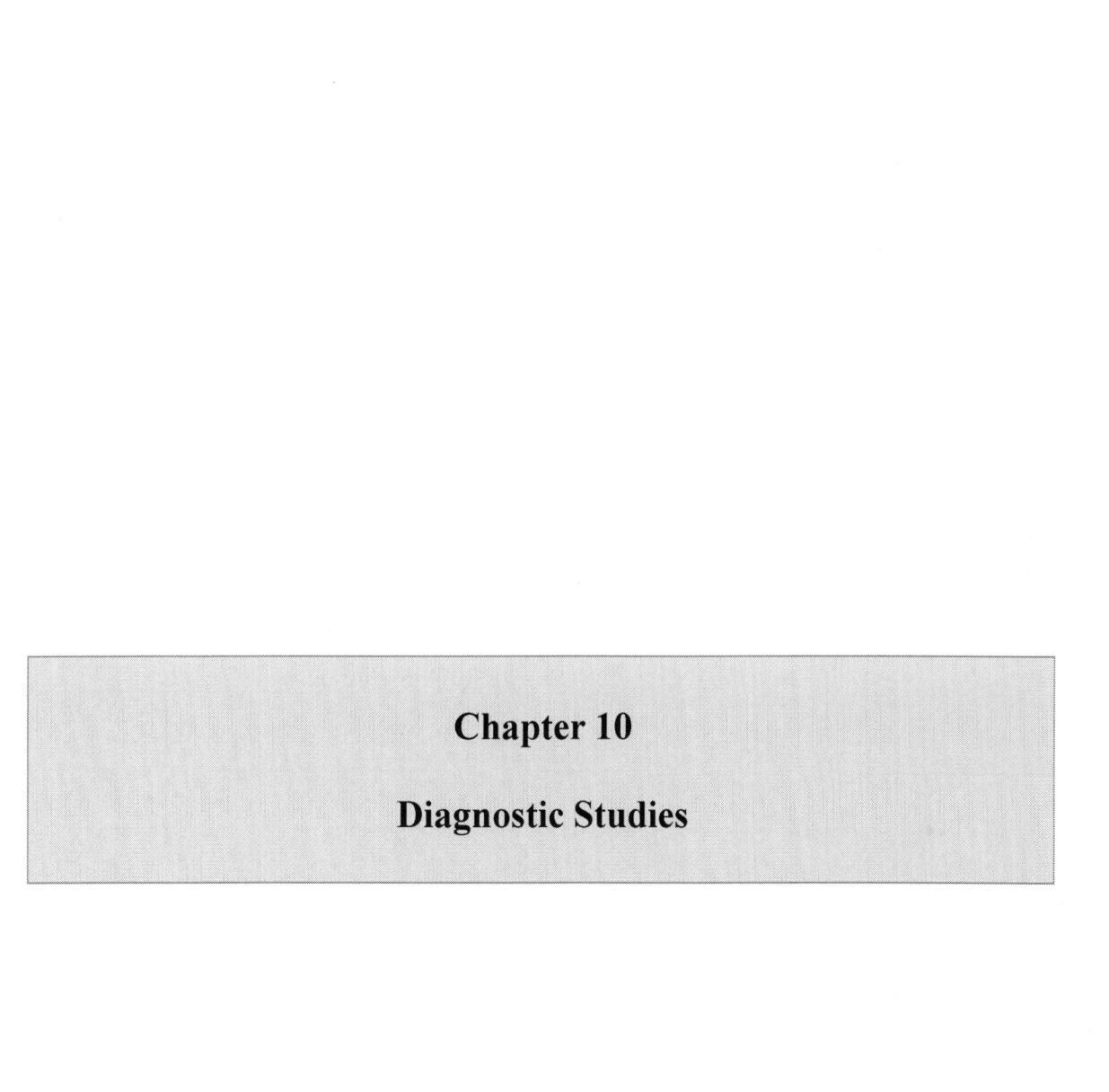

Diagnostic Studies

Chest X-ray

Front and side views are taken to determine the presence of cardiomegaly, pleural effusion, or congestive heart failure (an enlarged cardiac silhouette may suggest pericardial effusion).

NOTES

Echocardiography

A noninvasive study designed to confirm pericardial effusion (fluid), cardiac chamber enlargement, increased wall thickening, valvular heart disease, or volume overload.

NOTES

Electrocardiogram (ECG or EKG)

Electrodes are placed on the extremities and on the chest in specific locations. The conduction ability of the heart is measured and any abnormalities can be noted.

Note: In the dialysis patient, an elevated T wave is an indication of hyperkalemia.

NOTES

Fistulagram

Radiopaque dye is injected into the venous side of the access. A venous needle is placed in the fistula and the dye is injected. The path of the dye can then be traced by x-ray to determine any blockage or deviation in the vessel. If a blockage is found, angioplasty then is performed.

NOTES

Metabolic Bone Survey

X-ray of the hands and lumbar spine. Occasionally the feet are taken to check for bone demineralization.

NOTES

Nerve Conduction Study (NCS)

This procedure tests the conduction ability of the nerves in the extremities. A mild electrical current is passed through the muscle fibers and the response is measured. An electromylogram is a method of recording the electrical currents generated in an active muscle. An NCS is used to determine the presence and degree of peripheral neuropathy in the dialysis patient.

NOTES

*The man who has confidence in himself
gains the confidence of others.*

- Hasidic Saying

Chapter 11

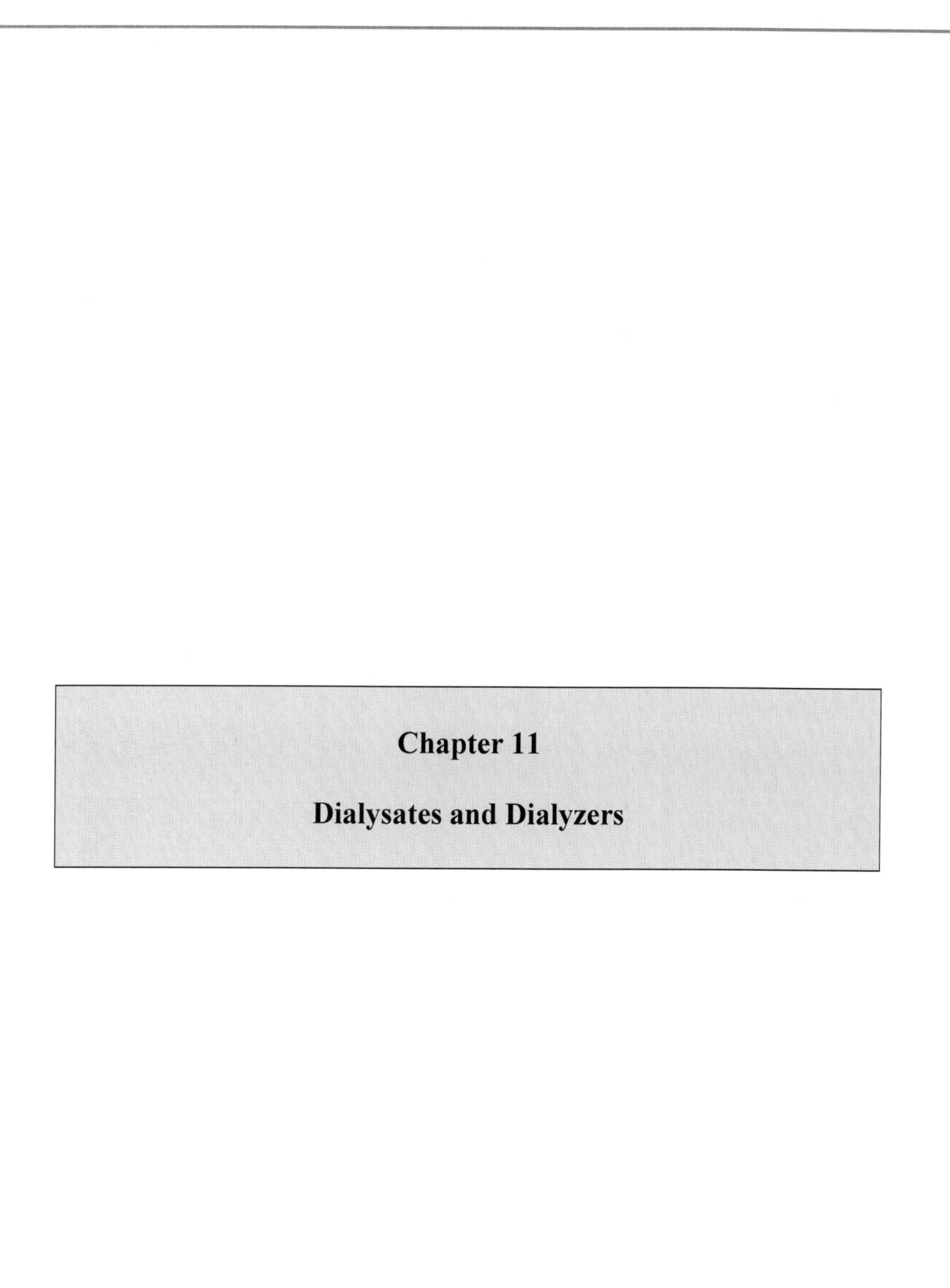

Dialysates and Dialyzers

Composition of Dialyzing Fluid

Five chemicals mixed with purified water are usually used: *

- Sodium chloride (NaCl)   135
- Sodium bicarbonate (NaHCO3)   37.0
- Calcium chloride (CaCl2)   3.5
- Potassium Chloride   2.0
- Magnesium chloride (MgCl2)   1.5

Approximate concentration (mEq/L) when 1 part is diluted with 34 parts of purified water. Please note that concentrations of these chemicals can be changed as per physician orders.

NOTES

| **Components of the Dialyzer** |

Most dialyzers are manufactured of four primary components:

- a. Blood compartment
- b. Dialyzing fluid compartment
- c. Semipermeable membrane
- g. Membrane-support structure

NOTES

| Coil | HISTORICAL |

The coil dialyzer contains one or two long tubes of cellulose membrane wrapped in a spiral fashion and supported by a rigid plastic mesh. The coil is submerged in a canister filled with dialyzing fluid (bath). Blood is introduced into the tube using a blood pump. The dialyzing fluid circulates easily around the coiled membrane and through the open mesh support structure.

The coil is a positive pressure dialyzer.

NOTES

HD (Hoeltzenbein)

HISTORICAL

The HD dialyzer contains multiple polystyrene membrane supports, each with a network of small grooves and ridges on one side. The side of each support is wrapped with cuprammonium cellulose. When the supports are packed together inside the dialyzer, the grooves and ridges press against the cuprammonium cellulose forming a capillary network in the membrane.

The HD is a negative pressure dialyzer.

NOTES

Hollow Fiber

This dialyzer stemmed from the development of a procedure to spin cellulose acetate into tiny hollow fibers. Thousands of fibers are encased in a clear plastic case. Blood is introduced into the fibers using a blood pump and dialysate is pumped around the fibers, with the fibers acting as the membrane. The hollow-fiber dialyzer may be reused several times if cleaned and store properly. *

This type of artificial kidney is a negative pressure dialyzer.

Law prohibits reuse without patient's signed consent.

NOTES

Parallel or Flat Plate

This type of dialyzer contains sheets of cellulose membrane sandwiched between rigid polypropylene plates. Dialysate is pumped into the space between the blood layers. The blood is pumped into the membrane by a blood pump.

This dialyzer is a negative pressure dialyzer.

NOTES

Believe in yourself!
Have faith in your abilities!
Without a humble but reasonable confidence in your powers you cannot be successful and happy.

- Norman Vincent Peale

Chapter 12

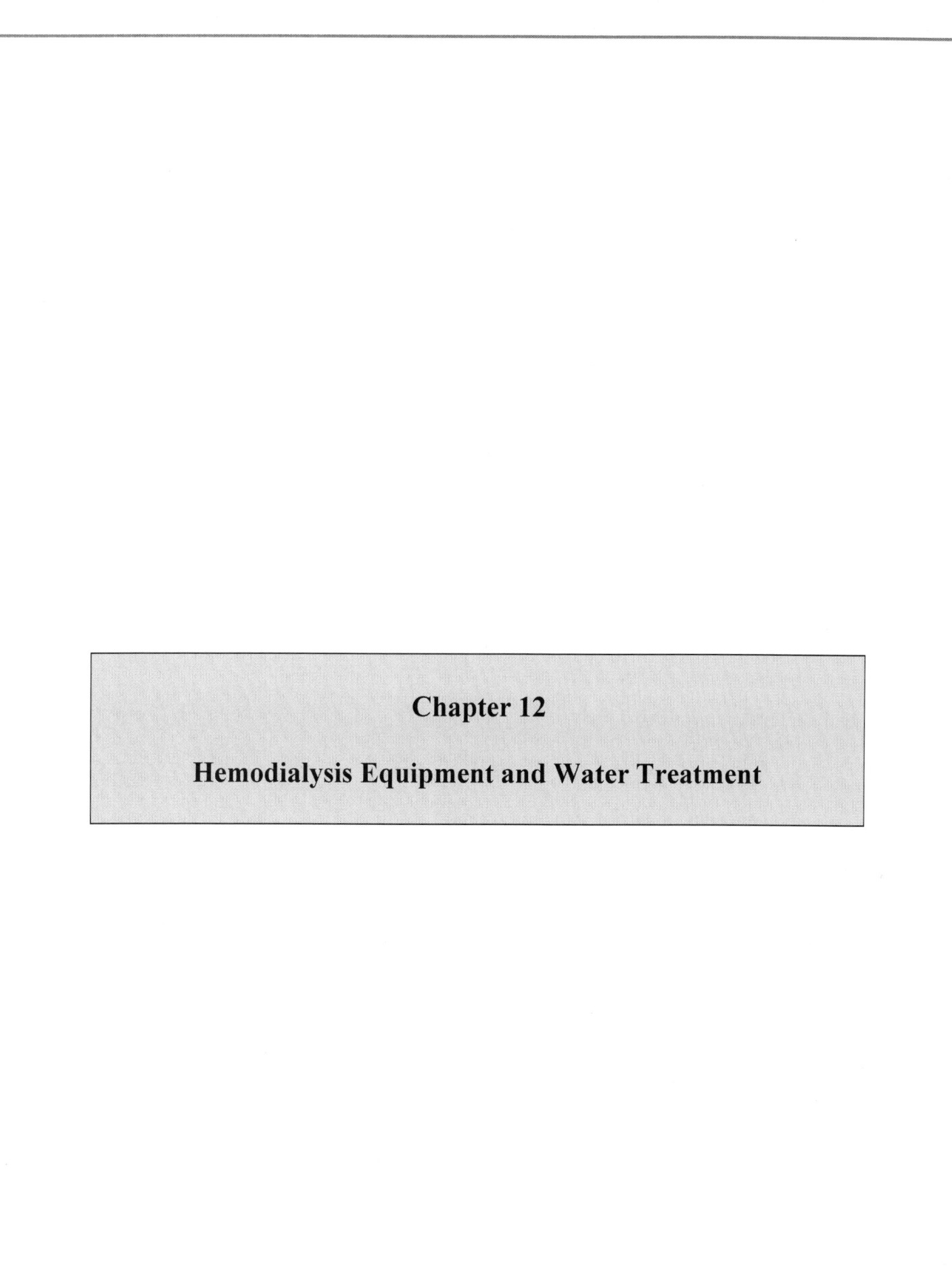

Hemodialysis Equipment and Water Treatment

Air Detector (Foam Detector, Air –Embolism Detector)

A device used for detection of air in the venous chamber, to prevent an air embolism. If air is detected, it will occlude the venous line, stop the blood pump, and trigger an audio alarm.

NOTES

Batch Delivery System | HISTORICAL

The delivery system has a reservoir in which dialyzing fluid could be prepared and stored for circulation to the dialyzer. The dialyzing solution is pumped up into the canister; it then recirculates through the dialyzer and back into the canister by another pump. This system is called a recirculating, single-pass system because of his two-stage process; the dialyzing fluid passes from the lower reservoir only once, but it passes through the upper canister numerous times.

Other Components

Temperature gauge, a mercoid switch for reading positive pressure, a heater, and a bath flow meter. No conductivity meter.

Example

Travenol RSP

NOTES

Bed-side Station (Central delivery system dependent) — HISTORICAL

The bed-side station is a more simple machine compared to a single station, since the dialysate is mixed and monitored by the central delivery system.

Other Components

Arterial and venous monitors, blood leak detector, dialysate flow meter. Some may have a temperature gauge and a canister or negative pressure pump, or both.

Example

Drake-Willock
Extracorporeal

NOTES

Blood Pump

The blood pump is used to circulate the patient's blood through the extra-corporeal system. The roller pump is most commonly used in clinical hemodialysis. The blood pump with a good AV access will move blood at 400cc/min.

NOTES

Central Delivery System — **HISTORICAL**

The central system was designed to deliver dialysate to bed-side stations. It mixes 34 parts of treated water to 1 part of concentrate. It has a conductivity meter that will put the machine on bypass if the concentration is out of limits. It will also alarm.

Other Components

Vacuum pump, heaters, bubble trap, alarm for high or low temperature.

Example

Drake-Willock
Extracorporeal

NOTES

Heparin Pump

The pump is used to infuse heparin during the hemodialysis treatment to prevent clotting of the extracorporeal blood. The heparin pump has an audio alarm to indicate that the syringe containing heparin is empty. It also has the ability to infuse at different rates.

It can also be used to infuse protamine sulfate in the venous line when doing regional heparinization.

NOTES

Proportioning Unit (Single patient)

This type of equipment mixes 34 parts of treated water and 1 part of concentrate. It has a built-in conductivity meter to identify the right concentration of dialysate. If for any reason the concentration changes, permitting the conductivity meter to move out of limits, the dialysate flow will go into bypass. The patient will not receive the wrong concentration. The machine will also alarm. This machine is a single pass, meaning fresh dialysate solution goes through the dialyzer only once.

Other Components

Vacuum pump, dialysate flow meter, heaters, bubble trap, arterial and venous monitors, blood leak detector, temperature gauge, negative pressure pump.

Example

Fresinius
Baxter
Cobe

NOTES

Single-needle Device

When only one access is available for hemodialysis (single-needle), this device is very helpful; it allows arterial blood and venous blood to circulate in and out on equal intervals.

The hemodialysis treatment using a single needle is not as efficient as using two accesses (i.e., two fistula needles) since blood recirculation occurs.

Example

Single-needle device by Hospal.

NOTES

Sorbsystem (Redy)

The only delivery system to utilize the advances of sorbent dialysate regeneration, Sorbsystem eliminates the need for special plumbing and water treatment; it requires only about six liters of water. The Sorbsystem cartridges will regenerate this water during the dialysis treatment. Using a layer of activated carbon, the cartridge also removes heavy metals and other substances found in untreated water.

Critical controls such as blood line pressure and conductivity are displayed on an electronic bar graph for adjustment and visibility. Acute, chronic, and home dialysis can be performed where and when it is needed.

Manufactured by Organon Teknika.

NOTES

Water Treatment

Different methods and combinations are used for hemodialysis:

a. Filtration
b. Softening
c. Distillation
d. Deionization
e. Adsorption by activated charcoal
f. Reverse osmosis (RO)

The Association for the Advancement of Medical Instrumentation has developed a set of standards to be use in treating water used in hemodialysis treatments. The standards are followed by dialysis units to maintain quality control. For further information or copies of the Standards, write to:

Association for the Advancement of Medical Instrumentation
1901 North Ft. Myer Drive, Suite 602
Arlington, Virginia 22209

NOTES

*There are admirable potentialities in every human being.
Believe in your strength and your youth.
Learn to repeat endlessly to yourself, "It all depends on me."*

- Andre Gide

Chapter 13

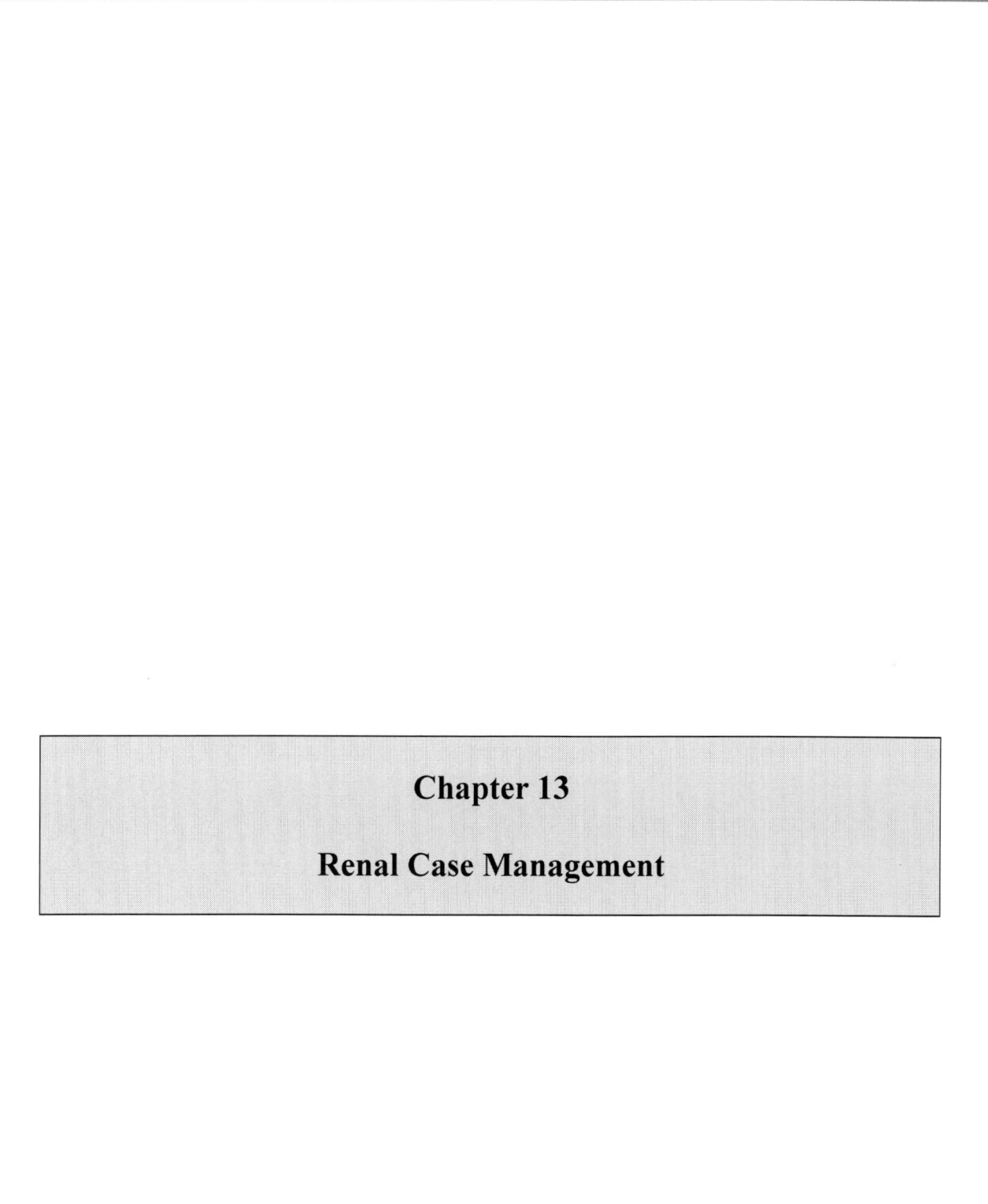

Renal Case Management

Renal Case Management

Defining case management

The definition of nursing case management varies depending on the discipline employed, the personnel and staff mix used, and the setting in which the model is implemented. Primarily borrowing principles from managed care systems, nursing case management is an approach that focuses on the coordination, integration, and direct delivery of patient services. It places internal controls on the resources used for care. Such management emphasizes early assessment and intervention, comprehensive care planning, and inclusive service system referrals.

The most effective means of managing this population is a field-based program using nurses to coordinate the care of the patients among the various medical providers they use. Although it is possible to have an impact on these very ill patients with a telephonic program, to achieve optimal results, there must be an onsite presence. An onsite presence makes it easier to assess patient needs and integrate with health plans and providers to streamline the delivery system for these patients. Improved patient and provider education and compliance leads to the elimination of unnecessary or inappropriate utilization of services.

NOTES

Renal Case Management

A sample team for Renal Case Management will have the following members:

- Physician - Nephrologist

- Renal Case Manager/Coordinator: Registered Nurse – Dialysis experience preferred

- Clinical Social Worker - Chronic Diseases experience

- Dietitian – Renal experience preferred

Some Teams may also have the following members:

- Pharmacist – Renal experience preferred

- Vascular Access Coordinator – Registered Nurse with Hemodialysis experience preferred

- Transplant Coordinator – Registered Nurse

NOTES
Other members you may think about to create the Renal Dream Team?

*Enthusiasm is the greatest asset in the world.
It beat money, power and influence.*

- Henry Chester

Chapter 14

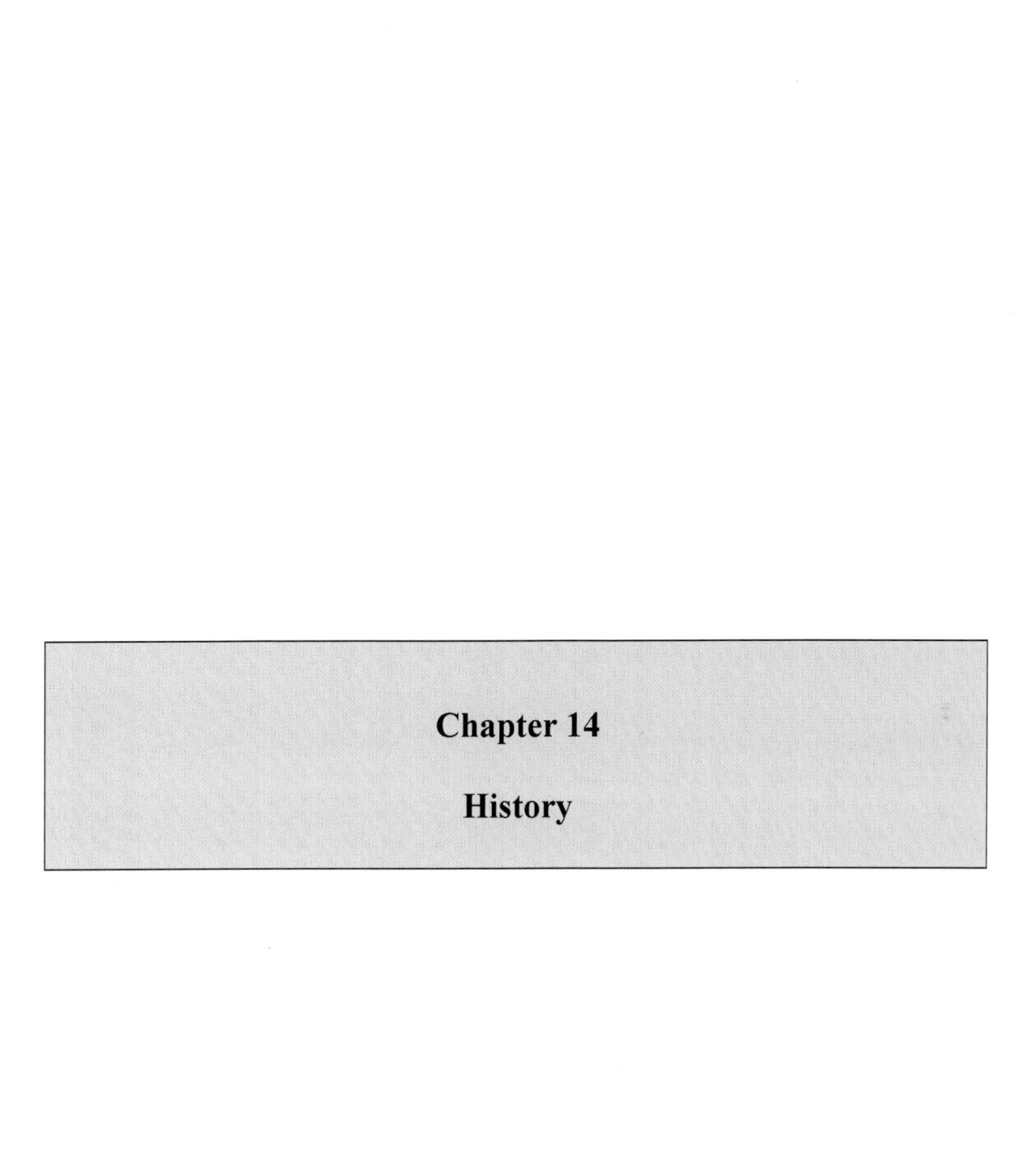

History

History

The following are brief markers in the history of hemodialysis:

1855   The German physiologist Adolph Fick had used collodion membranes in diffusion studies. A marked improvement over the parchment paper material previously employed in diffusion studies. The *selective* permeability of collodion remains an important characteristic of current dialyzer membranes that hold back substances with a molecular weight larger than 500 and clear the smaller toxins or solutes intended for removal.

1900   At Johns Hopkins University in Baltimore, John J. Abel, Leonard G. Rowntree and B. B. Turner begun to work actively on a dialyzer system and, in 1913, published their first article on the technique of "vividiffusion," or as we know it today, *hemodialysis*.

1914   Another group, working at the Pharmacological Laboratory, Northwestern University Medical School, Chicago, developed a unique diffusion device that it not required anticoagulants. The dialyzer operated on the principle of high blood flow, which was achieved by connection to the carotid artery.

1915   A German investigator, George Haas, used multiple dialyzers to increase the surface area of the semipermeable membrane, thereby exposing more blood to the dialyzing solution. He arranged as many as six cylinders in parallel to achieve the desire area, but arterial pressure was not great enough to propel blood through the entire apparatus. Haas therefore developed a rudimentary *blood pump* that consisted of a simple wheel and an electric motor.

Another investigator, Heinrich Necheles, working at University of Hamburg Medical School in Germany, was responsible for a very important feature incorporated into many contemporary dialyzers: the sandwiching of membrane material His technique was a significant improvement over Haas' method because it increased the surface area of the membrane without necessitating the use of more than one dialyzer.

1937   The German scientist Wilhelm Thalheimer discovered that a membrane used in sausage industry could be employed in removing solutes from the blood, This man-made cellulose acetate material (cellophane) was uniform in thickness, strong, and could be produced in large quantities. It was also inexpensive.

Willem Kolff, a young physician working at the University of Groningen in the Netherlands, was one of the first investigators to suggest that toxins might be removed from the blood of patients suffering renal failure.

1940 Kolff designed and built a number of artificial kidney machines using a rotating drum, which provided adequate surface area for human dialysis. Complete dialysis with the Kolff kidney required approximately six hours.

1950 Paul Teschan created a renal insufficiency center at the 11th Evacuation Hospital during the Korean War using a Kolff-Brigham kidney. This phase of Teechan's work is considered the forerunner of the multiple dialysis now used in treating patients suffering from chronic renal failure.

1956 The first commercially available, completely *disposable* dialyzer system designed and manufactured by Travenol Laboratories based on Kolff's kidney designed; the coil.

1960 The first A.V. shunt was implanted by Quinton and Scribner.

James Cimino developed the concept of the internal fistula. With the help of Michael Brescia were successful with the development of the internal fistula. This new access contributed greatly to the expansion of care for chronic renal patients, for it allowed continuous access to the blood stream without the danger of shunt disconnection or infection.

In the late 1950's Fredrik Kiil of Norway developed a parallel-plate dialyzer. It appears that Kiil was the first to use a new cellulose membrane called Cuprophane.

1961 Stanley Shaldon reported that his group at the Royal Free Hospital in London had successfully trained a patient to do home hemodialysis.

1967 Richard Stewart developed and tried clinically the first hollow-fiber dialyzer. The surface area was approximately one square meter.

*Education is what survives
when what has been learned has been forgotten.*

- B.F. Skinner

Chapter 15

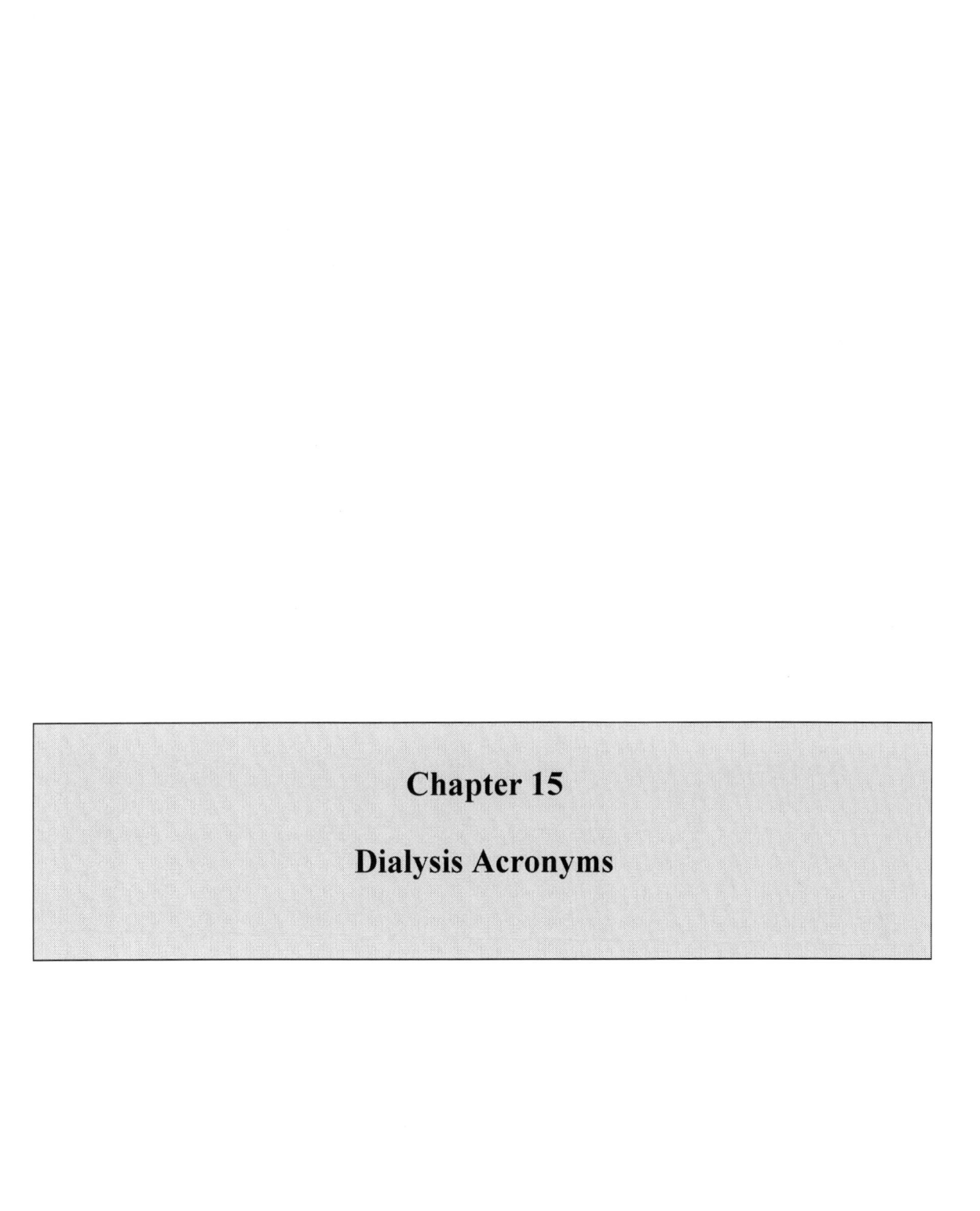

Dialysis Acronyms

DIALYSIS ACRONYMS

AAMI – See "Association for the Advancement of Medical Instrumentation"

ABDOMEN - The portion of the trunk located between the back, below the diaphragm, and including the lower portion of the abdominopelvic cavity. Contains the stomach, lower part of the esophagus small and large intestines, liver, gallbladder, spleen, pancreas, bladder.

ABSCESS – An abscess is a localized infection under the skin that looks like a blister or pimple filled with fluid or pus. If fistula needles are inserted into or near an abscess, infection of the fistula or graft or any other tissues may occur.

ACCESS – An access is a route into the blood stream that follows sufficient blood flow for hemodialysis. For a permanent vascular access, a vein is surgically connected to an artery, either directly (arteriovenous fistula) or with a piece of a synthetic tubing called a graft. For a temporary vascular access, a catheter must be inserted into a large central vein, such as the internal jugular vein in the neck. (*See also: Arteriovenous, Fistula, Catheter, and Graft*).

ACETATE - A salt of acetic acid.

ACID – Acid is a substance with a pH below 7.0 that is capable of donating a hydrogen ion (H+). In the human body, acids are created when protein and other substances are broken down by cell metabolism. Acids are salts, lemon juice, etc. (*See also Buffer, pH*).

ACIDOSIS - The hydrogen ion is increased thus the pH is decreased. A pathologic condition resulting from accumulation of acid or depletion of the alkaline reserve in the blood and body tissues.

ACQUIRED IMMUNODEFFICIENCY SYNDROME (AIDS) - See Human Immunodeficiency Virus (HIV).

ACUTE – Sudden onset. Having severe symptoms and a short course.

ACUTE RENAL FAILURE – Acute renal failure (ARF) is kidney failure with a sudden onset. An illness, injury, or toxin that stresses the kidneys usually causes it. In many cases of acute renal failure, patients who survive are able to recover their kidney function with temporary support provided by dialysis. In other cases, patients may develop chronic, irreversible renal failure.

ADSORB – To cause particles or molecules in a solution to stick to a surface of a solid material. To attract and retain other material on the surface.

ADVANCED DIRECTIVES – Advanced directives are documents that outline a patient's wishes for medical treatment or no treatment (comfort care only), in case the patient becomes too ill to make such decisions at a later date. A living will is an example of an advance directive. The patient's family members and other members of the health care team should be informed of the patient's wishes when an advanced directive has been prepared.

AIR DETECTOR – The air detector monitors blood in the venous line of the extra corporeal circuit for air. Air in the patient's blood stream can interfere with blood flow or heartbeat, causing death. If the air detector detects air, an alarm will sound, the blood pump will stop, and the venous bloodline will clamp to prevent air from reaching the patient.

AIR EMBOLISM – An air embolism occurs when air bubbles enter the bloodstream and are carried into a vessel small enough to be blocked by the air. In the vessel, the air embolus acts like a clot, blocking the flow of blood. Symptoms depend on the location of the air and the position of the patient. Dialysis machines have monitors to detect air in the venous bloodline to help prevent this potentially fatal complication.

ALBUMIN – Albumin is a blood protein that helps regulate osmotic pressure. Low serum albumin levels (<3.5 g/dl) may mean that a patient has malnutrition, which is very common in hemodialysis patients, and is linked to an increase of death. The presence of albumin in the urine indicates malfunction of the kidney, and may accompany kidney disease or heart failure. (*See also: Osmotic Pressure*).

ALKALOSIS - A pathologic condition resulting from accumulation of base, or from loss of acid without comparable loss of base in the body fluids.

ALUM – An aluminum compound often added to city water supplies to make the water clearer. Aluminum can build up in the bodies of the dialysis patients; therefore, it is important to keep the aluminum in the water used for dialysis at low levels by treating the water used to make dialysate.

ALUMINUM RELATED BONE DISEASE (ARBD) – ARBD is a bone disease caused by prolonged exposure to aluminum. Healthy kidneys secrete aluminum as waste. Aluminum builds up in the tissues at the point where new bone forms, can be seen on X-ray. Sources of aluminum include water used for dialysate, medications, and aluminum cookware. Aluminum based phosphate binders are also a source of exposure, but these have widely been replaced with calcium-based binders. The symptoms of ARBD can include deep bone pain, muscle weakness, and possible fractures.

AMYLOIDOSIS – Amyloidosis is a disorder thought to result from building-up in the body of a starch-like protein (called beta 2- microglobulin) normally removed by healthy kidneys. This protein is almost insoluble and once it infiltrates the tissues they become waxy and nonfunctioning. The protein is believed to accumulate in the bones, joints, and other tissues of some renal patients, causing arthritis-like joint pain, and/or bone pain. The use of high flux dialysis membrane can remove the beta 2- microglobulin associated with amyloidosis, which may help prevent or treat this disorder.

ANAPHYLACTIC REACTION – An anaphylactic reaction, or anaphylaxis, is an immediate severe reaction to a substance to which an individual is allergic. The reaction may include hives, itching, or wheezing; the reaction may develop into anaphylactic shock, causing hypotension, cardiac arrhythmias, or asystole, spasms of breathing passages, and swelling of the throat can even cause death.

ANASTOMOSIS – Communication between two vessels. An anastomosis is a surgical connection. In a hemodialysis access, a connection is made between blood vessels – as in a vein and an artery connected to form an arteriovenous fistula. dialysis needles should not be inserted directly into an area of the anastomosis.

ANATOMY - The structure of an organism. The branch of science dealing with the form and structure of organisms.

ANEMIA – Anemia is a shortage of oxygen-carrying red blood cells. Because red blood cells bring oxygen to all the cells in the body, anemia causes severe fatigue, heart disorders, difficulty concentrating, reduced immune function, and other problems. Anemia is common among renal patients, caused by insufficient erythropoietin, iron deficiency, repeated blood losses, and other factors. Anemia is treated with EPOGEN (Epoitin Alfa), a synthetic form of erythropoietin, and with iron supplements. (*See also: EPOGEN, Erythropoietin, Hematocrit, and Hemoglobin*).

ANESTHETIC – An anesthetic is a drug that numbs the body to prevent pain. Local anesthetics can be injected into a certain spot (such as into the skin around a puncture site before needle insertion), or applied to the skin to prevent pain at the site.

ANEURYSM – An aneurysm is a ballooning or bulging of a weak spot in a blood vessel. Because the aneurysm can rupture, or burst causing severe bleeding great care must be taken in a patient who has one. Aneurysms can occur if needles are inserted too often into the same area of the fistula.

ANION – Ion carrying a negative electric charge.

ANGIOPLASTY – Angioplasty is a medical procedure used to dilate, or open up, a narrowed area of a blood vessel, called a stenosis. In dialysis patients, Angioplasty may be used to treat a stenosis in a vascular access. A small balloon is treated through the blood vessel into the access and gently inflated to push the walls of the vessel open.

ANTEROGRADE – Anterograde means with the direction of flow. With a fistula or graft, the anterograde flow is the needle pointing away from the anastomosis. (Retrograde means against the flow and the needle tip must be 1 inch away from the anastomosis). The venous needle is always placed anterograde while the arterial needle can be placed anterograde or retrograde in the vascular access.

ANTICOAGULANT – A medication or chemical that prevents clotting of the blood. Any substance that in vivo or in vitro suppresses, delays, or nullifies coagulation of the blood. In dialysis patients, anticoagulants, such as heparin, are used to prevent formation of blood clots in the extra corporeal circuit during hemodialysis *(See also: Heparin)*.

ANTIDIURETIC HORMONE (ADH) – Antidiuretic hormone, or vasopressin, is released by the pituitary gland in the brain. ADH triggers the normal kidneys to reabsorb more water, to help prevent excess fluid loss. Vasopressin also triggers the blood vessels to constrict or tighten.

ANTISEPTICS - Antiseptics are products that stop or interfere with the growth of bacteria or viruses. They are used to kill microorganisms, to prevent infection and the spread of disease. *(See also: Microorganisms)*.

ANTITHROMBOGENIC - Prevents the formation of clots.

APICAL PULSE - The apical pulse is the pulse felt on the chest wall directly over the heart.

APNEA - Apnea is the temporary period when breathing stops due to various causes. The prefix "A" before the word means without. Pnea means breathing. In obstructive apnea there is respiratory effort but no air flows because of upper airway obstruction.

ARRHYTHMIA - An arrhythmia is an irregularity of the heartbeat, which may be felt as irregular pulses or heard directly over the heart. Also called dsyrythmia. (Without rhythm).

ARTERIAL PRESSURE - In dialysis, arterial pressure is measured within the arterial drip chamber, between the patient's arterial needle and the blood pump – as pre-pump arterial pressure. (Can also be measured as post pump pressure – after the blood pump and before the dialyzer).

ATERIAL PRESSURE MONITOR - The arterial pressure is measured in the arterial drip chamber and there is a pressure monitor line connected to a transducer protector. The transducer takes the pressure and gives a read out on the monitor (a gauge or screen). The pressure is usually a pre pump blood pressure and is therefore a negative pressure because the blood pump is pulling blood from the patient's vascular access. A positive pressure is when the drip chamber pressure reading is post blood pump. (See *also: Extracorporeal Circuit*).

ARTERIALIZED - In creation of an AV fistula, the blood from the artery anastomosed to a vein crosses over, dilates and thickens the vein.

ARTERIOVENOUS (AV) FISTULA - A fistula is an opening between body and cavities. In people with renal failure, an arteriovenous fistula is a surgical connection between and artery and a vein. Just beneath the skin of the arm or leg. Dr. James Cimino and Dr. James Brecia developed the surgery in 1966. In an AV fistula, a strong flow of arterial blood is shunted to a vein. The force of the blood flowing from the artery thickens the vein wall. A mature fistula can be punctured repeatedly with dialysis needles and provide the rapid blood flow rates needed for dialysis.

ARTERY - An artery is a blood vessel that carries blood away from the heart at high pressure. Arteries deliver oxygenated blood to every part of the body. Arteries have muscles in their walls and veins have valves.

ARTIFICIAL – Artificial means man made, usually in imitation of something found in nature. The dialyzer is often called an artificial kidney, because it is a synthetic piece of equipment that imitates the function of a kidney.

ASCITES - Ascites is a build up of fluid in the abdomen caused by liver damage, and heart failure, malnutrition or infection. Special ultrafiltration procedures and other methods (i.e. abdominal drainage) may be required to remove the excess fluid.

ASEPSIS - Asepsis is the absence of disease producing microorganisms. Asepsis in dialysis is accomplished by disinfection, maintaining dialysis equipment, and using aseptic technique for invasive procedures, such as inserting dialysis needles.

ASEPTIC – Aseptic means germ-free, or sterile.

ASSOCIATION FOR THE ADVANCEMENT OF MEDICAL INSTRUMENTATION --- Develops <u>voluntary</u> standards for various aspects of dialysis treatment, including maximum levels of water contamination and methods of dialyzer processing.

AUSCULTATION – Auscultation means listening with a stethoscope. Auscultation of a patient's vascular access is used to help diagnose problems like stenosis or thrombosis that can change the normal sound of the bruit.

BACKFILTRATION – Back filtration is movement of dialysate across the dialyzer membrane into the patient's blood. It can be caused by a change in the pressure or concentration gradient between dialysate and blood. Backfiltration may be more likely to occur with high flux dialyzer membranes, which have larger pores, and thus are more permeable. Backfiltration can be dangerous to the patient because endotoxins contained in non-sterile dialysate can enter the bloodstream directly causing congestive heart failure. *(See also: Permeable).*

BACKWASHING – Backwashing means forcing water backward through a filter. This technique can be used to remove accumulated particles from clogged sediment filters in a water treatment system. *(See also: Filters).*

BACTERIA – Plural for bacterium. Bacteria are microscopic, single-cell organisms that can cause disease. Bacteria are classified as gram-positive or gram-negative by the color they turn on a standard laboratory test called Gram's stain. *(See also: Endotoxin, Gram-negative, Gram-positive).*

BASE - Base is a chemical that is capable of accepting a hydrogen ion (H+). A substance with a pH of greater than 7.0 is considered to be a base, alkali. In the body, bicarbonate is a base. In the chemical processes of the body, bases are essential to the maintenance of a normal acid-base balance.

BICARBONATE - Bicarbonate is a buffer found in the blood that is reabsorbed by health kidneys. Bicarbonate is used by the body to neutralize acids formed when protein and other foods are metabolized. Patients with kidney failure can no longer secrete hydrogen ions and can no longer regulate or reabsorb enough bicarbonate to replenish blood supplies. As a result, these patients cannot neutralize acids very well, so bicarbonate is most commonly used in dialysate to help restore levels of bicarbonate in the body. Bicarbonate buffer has the advantage of being quickly used by the body, making dialysis more comfortable for the patients. The main disadvantage of using bicarbonate dialysate are its ability to support bacterial growth, and the need for two separate dialysate concentrates (acid and bicarbonate) to prevent the formation of precipitate (calcium carbonate or magnesium), that can interfere with the normal operation of dialysis equipment. (*See also: Buffer*).

BIOCOMPATIBLE - Means similar to the human body—and thus less likely to cause adverse immune responses normally triggered by a foreign "invader". Some dialyzer membrane materials (such as polysulfone) are considered more biocompatible than cellulose membranes. However cellulose membranes can become more compatible after use. A coating of blood protein develops inside a cellulose dialyzer after it has been used tricking the patient's immune system treating the membrane as less "foreign". (*See also: Cellulose*).

BLOOD LEAK – A blood leak occurs when the delicate semipermeable membrane of the dialyzer tears, allowing blood to leak into the dialysate. Severe blood leaks can cause major blood loss during dialysis (Keep in mind that if the blood leaks out, dialysate can enter the bloodstream, which could cause bacteria to enter the patients blood).

BLOOD LEAK DETECTOR – Blood leak detector is an alarm system on the hemodialysis delivery system that monitors used dialysate for blood that would indicate a leak in the dialyzer membrane. Since a triggered alarm would stop the blood pump and the venous line clamps, this is a blood compartment alarm – even though it examines used dialysate. The detector shines a beam of light through the used dialysate into a photocell. Any break in the transmission of the light beam caused by (microscopic) blood cells will trigger the alarm. *(See also: Hemodialysis Delivery System)*.

BLOOD PATH - Conduit through which the blood passes. In dialysis, the arterial and venous sets and blood passages within the dialyzer make up a continuous extracorporeal blood path.

BLOOD PUMP - The blood pump is the part of the dialysis delivery system that moves the patient's blood through the extracorporeal circuit using a roller pump at a fixed rate of speed. During hemodialysis, the blood tubing is treaded between the pump head and the rollers. The rollers move blood through the extracorporeal circuit and back to the patient.

BLOOD PRESSURE - Blood pressure is a measurement of the amount of pressure exerted against the wall of vessels. The systolic blood pressure raises during activity or excitement and falls during sleep. The average blood pressure for a relaxed sitting adult is 120/80. Blood pressure varies with age, sex, altitude, muscular development, and according to states of mental and physical stress and fatigue. The blood pressure is determined by several interrelated factors, including the pumping action of the heart, the resistance to the flow of blood in the arterioles, the elasticity of the walls of the main arteries, the blood volume and extracellular fluid volume, and the blood viscosity, or thickness.

BLOOD PUMP SEGMENT- The blood pump segment is durable, larger diameter section of the arterial blood tubing that is threaded through the roller mechanism of the blood pump.

BLOOD TUBING (OR BLOODLINES) – Blood tubing is a part of the extracorporeal circuit that transports blood from the patient's vascular access through the arterial puncture site, to and from the dialyzer back to the patient through the venous tubing. There are two segments of blood tubing, the *arterial* (often color-coded red) and *venous* (often color-coded blue). Components of the blood tubing include patient connectors; dialyzer connectors, drip chamber/bubble trap, as well as the blood pump segment, and heparin and saline infusion lines.

BLOOD UREA NITROGEN - Urea is a waste product of protein metabolism, measured as blood urea nitrogen (BUN). Because patients with renal failure cannot remove urea from their body, it builds up between treatments and must be removed by dialysis. BUN is easily measured, so it is used as a stand in for other wastes that also build up in the blood between treatments but are difficult to identify. Measurement of BUN is the basis of kinetic modeling and urea reduction ration, methods for determining the adequacy of the dialysis treatment. (*See also: Hemodialysis Adequacy, Urea Kinetic Modeling, Urea Reduction Ratio, and Uremia*).

BOWMAN'S CAPSULE - The renal or malpighian corpuscle. It consists of a visceral layer closely applied to the glomerulus and an outer parietal layer. It functions as a filter in the formation of urine.

BRACHIAL PULSE - The brachial pulse felt at the brachial artery, in the crease of the elbow. The main artery of the arm.

BRACHIOCEPHALIC FISTULA - A brachiocephalic fistula is the most common type of fistula of the upper arm. The fistula is created by surgically joining the brachial artery and the cephalic vein. (*See also: Arteriovenous Fistula*).

BRUIT - (French word pronounced brew-ee) A bruit is a swooshing or buzzing sound caused by the high pressure flow of blood through the patient's AV fistula or graft. The bruit can be heard through a stethoscope at the anastomosis, and for some distance along the access. A low pitch bruit with both a systolic and diastolic component indicates a blood flow sufficient to permit dialysis. A high-pitch bruit may indicate stenosis of the access. [Many times a distinctive pulse instead of swooshing sound also indicates clotting of the graft/fistula may occur]. (aneurysmal bruit is a blowing sound heard over an aneurysm).

BUBBLE TRAP – See Drip Chamber.

BUFFER - A buffer is a substance that maintains the pH of a solution at constant level, despite the addition of acid or base. Bicarbonate and acetate are two buffers used in dialysis to maintain the pH of dialysate. (*See also: Acid, Bicarbonate*).

BUN – See Blood Urea Nitrogen.

BURETTE - A graduated glass tube used to deliver a measured amount of liquid.

BYPASS – Bypass is a safety feature of the hemodialysis delivery system that cuts off the flow of fresh dialysate to the dialyzer and shunts it to the drain. Bypass prevents unsafe dialysate (wrong conductivity, temperature, or pH) from reaching the patient and causing harm. (*See also: Hemodialysis Delivery System*).

CALCITRIOL – Calcitriol is the activated form of Vitamin D, produced by healthy kidneys, which is needed by the body to absorb calcium from food. Many dialysis patients need calcitriol supplements to turn off the PTH and to help avoid secondary hyperparathyroidism and bone disease. (*See also: Secondary Hyperthyroidism*).

CALCIUM – Calcium is an element that exists as a cation (positively charged ion) that is partly bond to protein in the blood. In the human body, calcium is an electrolyte needed for nerve and muscle function and normal bone formation. Too much or too little calcium in dialysate feed water supply can cause serious complications for the patients, including death. Calcium in a dialysis feed water supply can combine with other substances to form precipitate or scale that can clog dialysis machinery if bicarbonate buffered dialysate is used. Patient blood levels of calcium are usually checked monthly. (*See also: Electrolyte, Hypercalcemia, and Hypocalcemia*).

CANNULA - A tube that is inserted into an opening in the body. See: Shunt.

CAPD – See Continuous Ambulatory Peritoneal Dialysis.

CAPILLARIES - Capillaries are the body's smallest blood vessels, where blood crosses arteries to veins. Capillaries are even smaller in diameter that human hair; blood cells must line up single file to pass through. Unlike arteries and veins, capillary walls are semipermeable, allowing oxygen, food, and waste products to pass through. In the kidneys the glomerulus is a tiny ball of capillaries that filters out wastes, small essential solutes, and water from the blood because they are small enough to go through the selective glomerular membrane.

CARBON TANK – Carbon tanks are water treatment devices that contain granular activated carbon that absorbs molecular weight particles from water. Carbon tanks are used primarily to remove chlorine, chloramines, pesticides, and some trace organic substances from water used in dialysis.

CARDIAC ARREST – Cardiac arrest is a situation which the heart stops beating. Cardiac arrest can be a lethal side effect of certain dialysis incidents, such as the use of too warm dialysate, improper dialysate concentration, hemolysis, loss of too much blood, or a large amount of air entering the patient's blood stream. Hyperkalemia also can cause cardiac arrest. Synonyms that you need to know: asystole (without heartbeat), cardiac standstill, flat line (*See Also: Hemolysis and Hyperkalemia*).

CARDIAC OUTPUT - Cardiac output is the amount of blood passing through the heart in a certain period of time. The presence of an AV fistula or graft causes a 10% increase in the size of the heart. Patients who cannot tolerate this change in cardiac output are not good candidates for AV fistulae or grafts. (*See also: Arteriovenous Fistula*).

CARDIAC TAMPONADE - Cardiac Tamponade is a condition resulting from pericarditis (an accumulation of fluid in the pericardial sac) where the heart cannot beat accurately due to the fluid in the pericardial sac.

CARPAL TUNNEL SYNDROME - Paresthesias, pain, or numbness affecting some part of the median nerve distribution of the hand(s), i.e., palmar side of thumb, index finger, and radial half of the ring finger, and radial half of the palm. The parethesias and pain may radiate into the arm. There may be a history of cumulative trauma to the wrist, e.g, in carpenters, rowers, or those who regularly use vibrating tools or machinery.

CAPILLARY FLOW - A term used to describe a type of parallel-flow dialyzer in which the blood flows through tiny capillary-like tubes made of a semipermeable membrane. The mechanism by which a liquid rises in small tubes or fibers.

CATABOLISM – Catabolism is a complex chemical process in which substances (e.g., proteins) are broken down into simpler substances in the blood, producing waste products. The opposite of anabolism. Healthy kidneys normally remove these wastes (e.g. urea), but in dialysis patients, it must be removed during dialysis treatment.

CATHETER - A catheter is a plastic tube. In hemodialysis, a catheter is used to create a temporary or longer-term dialysis access. Catheters are often temporary or permanently implanted into the internal jugular vein (neck), femoral vein (groin), or subclavian vein (chest). The internal jugular and femoral sites are less likely than subclavian sites to cause central venous stenosis, a complication that can reduce the number of potential access sites the patient has. For this reason, NKF-DOQI guidelines recommend use of the internal jugular for hemodialysis catheters, when possible. In peritoneal dialysis, a catheter is surgically placed in the abdomen to allow fresh dialysate to be infused into the peritoneal cavity and used dialysate to be drained. (*See also: Central Venous Stenosis, Peritoneal Dialysis*).

CATION - A cation is a positively charged ion. In water treatment, cations can be removed by ion exchange or reverse osmosis water treatment to ensure acceptable contents of water used for dialysate and reprocessing. (*See also: Deionizer, Ion*).

CCPD – See continuous Cycling Peritoneal Dialysis.

CELL - A mass of protoplasm containing a nucleus or nucleal material. It is the unit of structure of all animals and plants. The basic structural unit of living organisms. All living cells arise from other cells, either by division or by fusion.

CELLULOSE – Cellulose is a fiber that forms the cell walls of plants. Cellulose acetate was the first material used as a dialyzer membrane by Dr. Willem Kolff in 1942. In water treatment, cellulose acetate was also the first material used to form reverse osmosis membranes. To form a membrane, cellulose can be dissolved in a solution containing copper salts and ammonium. The resulting material is formed into sheet of hollow fibers using a solution-spinning technique. Cellulose dialyzer membranes are the most likely to cause first-use syndrome in some patients, because of this they are not considered biocompatible. (*See also: Biocompatible, First-Use Syndrome*).

CENTRAL VENOUS STENOSIS - Central venous stenosis is a narrowing of the central veins of the body that can make the arm on the affected side of unsuitable for a vascular access. With a limited number of potential vascular access sites available in the human body, it is important to preserve as many as possible. High rates of central venous stenosis are the reason that the subclavian vein is not recommended by the NKF-DOQI guidelines for hemodialysis catheter placement.

CFU - See colony forming units.

CHLORAMINES - Chloramines are substances formed by mixing chlorine and ammonia, or created in nature when chlorine combines with organic material. Ammonia is added to municipal water supplies to boost the germ killing power of chlorine. Chlorine is an oxidant, a substance that destroys microorganisms by breaking their cell walls. If chloramines contaminate dialysis water, they can cause a serious condition called hemolysis (rupture of red blood cells) in patients. Carbon tanks are used to remove chloramines from water use for dialysis. (*See also: Carbon Tank*).

CHLORIDE – Chloride is a salt concentrate needed in dialysate and in the human body. Chloride combines with other elements to form sodium chloride, potassium chloride, magnesium chloride, and calcium chloride.

CHLORINE - The element chlorine is a greenish-yellow gas that can cause severe irritation to the lungs if inhaled. Chlorine is combined with other ingredients (such as in sodium hypochlorite-bleach) to disinfect surfaces. Chlorine may also be added to the municipal water supplies to destroy microorganisms. Carbon tanks are used to remove chlorine and chloramines from water used for hemodialysis and the dialyzer reuse.

CHRONIC RENAL FAILURE (CRF) - Chronic means ongoing, continuing, or long-term. Chronic renal failure is a long, usually slow process that involves progressive loss of nephrons, and thus loss of kidney function. Chronic renal failure can take many years and may not cause symptoms until advanced stage. End-stage renal disease (ESRD) is an endpoint of chronic renal failure; if refers to the point at which renal replacement therapy (e.g. dialysis) is required for survival. (*See also: End Stage Renal Disease, Nephrons*).

CLEARANCE (K) - Clearance is a quantity of blood (in ml) that is completely cleared of a solute in one minute of dialysis at a given blood flow rate and dialysate rate. Clearance is a measure of dialyzer performance, and is one of the characteristics of dialyzers that can affect the dialysis effectiveness. Manufactures often test dialyzers with solutions other than blood (in vitro), so actual clearance of a given dialyzer during dialysis (in vivo) can vary significantly from the manufacturer's stated clearance. Mathematical expression of the rate at which a given substance is removed from a solution. (*See also: Hemodialysis Adequacy*).

CLINICAL PRACTICE GUIDELINES - Clinical practice guidelines are recommendations for patient care developed by expert panels and/or by a thorough review of medical literature. The National Kidney Foundation-Dialysis Outcomes Quality Initiative (NKF-DOQI) guidelines released in 1997 cover four key areas of Nephrology: Anemia, hemodialysis adequacy, peritoneal dialysis adequacy, and vascular access. The goal of the NKF-DOQI clinical practice guidelines is to improve patient outcomes. (*See also: Patient Outcomes*).

COEFFICIENT OF ULTRAFILTRATION (KUF) - The kuf is the fixed amount of fluid that a dialyzer will remove from the patient's blood per hour, at a specified pressure. The kuf is also called the ultrafiltration factor (UFF) or ultrafiltration rate (UFR) and is expressed in milliliters (ml) per hour (hr) of water removed for each millimeter (mm) of mercury (hg) of transmembrane pressure (TMP), or ml/hr/mm/Hg TMP. The higher the KUF, the more fluid per millimeter of mercury pressure will be removed. High-flux and high-efficiency dialyzers have higher kuf's than conventional dialyzers. Any KUF above 8 requires the use of volumetric control hemodialysis systems to precisely control the amount of fluid removed.

COLONY FORMING UNITS- The number of colony forming units (CFU) in a water or dialysate unit is measured by the number of living (able to form colonies) bacteria.

COMPOSITE RATE REIMBURSEMENT SYSTEM - A composite rate reimbursement system is a method of U.S Government payment for dialysis treatment. Dialysis facilities are paid a fixed, limited amount of money for each dialysis treatment given to a patient. The limited amount, the composite rate, must cover nearly all the services to dialysis patients.

CONCENTRATION - Concentration is the amount of solute(s) (i.e., potassium, sodium) dissolved in a measured amount of fluid (i.e., water, blood) A highly concentrated solution had more solutes and less fluid. The urine is concentrated, so that the proper amounts of fluid and other substances are retained in the body. In dialysis, the concentration of each of the substances in dialysate must be correct, to ensure a safe and effective procedure.

CONCENTRATON GRADIENT - See Gradient.

CONDUCTIVE SOLUTE TRANSFER - See diffusion.

CONDUCTIVITY - Conductivity is the ability of a solution to conduct electricity. It is a measure of ions in solution. A conductivity meter measures the electrolyte composition (or how many ions in a solution) of dialysate by measuring the dialysate's ability to conduct an electrical current; to be sure it is within the safe limit. Capacity for conductance.

CONDUCTIVITY ALARM – The conductivity alarm indicates an inappropriate mixture of water and dialysate concentrate. If this alarm has triggered, the dialysis machine will go into bypass mode, shunting dialysate to the drain.

CONFIDENTIALITY - Confidentiality is maintaining patient privacy. Patient information should be shared with the rest of the dialysis team when it is medically necessary. Patient information should not be shared outside the dialysis facility, or with other patients or visitors within or outside the facility.

CONGESTIVE HEART FAILURE (CHF) - Congestive heart failure occurs when the heart cannot pump out all the blood it receives, so that excess fluid backs up into the lungs. Fluid overload caused by too much fluid intake or not removing enough fluid during dialysis can lead to congestive heart failure. S/S: SOB/dyspnea and +4 leg/ankle/foot edema, have the patient turn their head to the side and look for distended neck veins.

CONTAMINATE - Substance or organisms that stains or soils and makes unfit for use.

CONTINUOUS AMBULATORY PERITONEAL DIALYSIS (CAPD) - CAPD is a form of peritoneal dialysis that can be done while the patient does his or her usual daily activities. Dialysate enters the patient's peritoneum through a catheter. The dialysate is allowed to remain in the patient's abdomen for a period of time (dwell), and then fresh dialysate is exchanged for used dialysate. Usually four to five exchanges are performed each day. Because dialysis occurs continuously, the patient's blood does not build up large amounts of wastes between treatments; the diet and fluids are less restricted that for hemodialysis patients. (*See also: Peritoneal Dialysis*).

CONTINUOUS CYCLING PERITONEAL DIALYSIS (CCPD) - CCPD can be learned after the patient has mastered CAPD. CCPD uses a machine "cycler" to put fluid into the patient's abdomen and drain in out at prescribed periods of time. The process is repeated with fresh dialysate for 8 too 12 hours, usually while the patient sleeps. The last exchange must be left in the abdomen, so the patient can continue to dialyze all day. (*See also: Peritoneal Dialysis*).

CONTINUOUS QUALITY IMPROVEMENT- CQI is a management theory based on the idea of constant improvement beyond the status quo. To be successful, all employees and administrators must use a philosophy of constant improvement. CQI often includes a cycle of planning procedures, implementing them, and checking performance (Plan-Do-Check-Act). In dialysis CQI can be a powerful tool for improving patient care.

CONTINUOUS RENAL REPLACEMENT THERAPY (CRRT) - CRRT is a form of extracorporeal therapy that uses either the patient's own heart or a pump to remove blood through an extracorporeal circuit. Usually CRRT is done continuously over many hours to very gently remove extra fluid and some wastes in patients to ill or too unstable for regular hemodialysis (usually in ICU) A cartridge containing a semipermeable membrane (Similar to a hemodialyzer is used).

CONFECTION, CONVECTIVE SOLUTE TRANSFER - See solute drag.

CONVENTIONAL DIALYSIS - Conventional dialysis uses a dialyzer with an invitro KUF below 6 to remove wastes and excess fluid from the patients with renal failure. Conventional dialysis treatments often take between 4 and 5 hours to achieve adequate dialysis. (*See also: Coefficient or Ultrafiltration, In Vivo*).

CUPRAMMONIUM PROCESS - Technique for producing regenerated cuprammonium cellulose membrane using an ammoniacal copper solution.

COUNTERCURRENT FLOW - A countercurrent flow within a dialyzer occurs when blood moves in one direction and dialysate flows in the opposite direction during dialysis. Countercurrent flow allows for the most efficient dialysis, because it keeps the blood in constant contact with fresh dialysate. Also known as flow geometry.

CREATININE - Creatinine is a waste product of creatinine and creatinine phosphate, an energy-storing molecule in the muscles normally excreted in urine. Creatinine is produced in proportion to muscle mass, that is, larger people with more muscle mass have higher creatinine levels. Since creatinine is normally produced in fairly constant amounts as a result of the breakdown of phosphocreatine and is excreted in the urine, an elevation in the creatinine level in the blood indicates a disturbance in kidney function.

CREATININE CLEARANCE - Creatinine clearance is a urine test that measures the kidney's ability to remove creatinine and other wastes from the blood. As chronic renal failure progresses, creatine clearance will fall to 10% of normal or less. (*See also: Chronic Renal Failure*).

CRENATION - Crenation is a shriveling of blood cell that occurs if the blood cells are exposed to a solution more concentrated than blood. For example, crenation may occur if dialysate with too much concentrate and not enough water is used (hypertonic solution) if crenation occurs, the blood will appear dark red. The condition can be fatal.

CUFFED-TUNNELED CATHETERS - Cuffed tunneled catheters are permanent dialysis catheters that are inserted into a blood vessel through a tunnel created under the patient's skin. Inside the tunnel tract, surround tissue grows into an attached cuff to help stabilize the catheter and provide a physical barrier to bacteria.

CYANOSIS - Cyanosis is the condition of having bluish-colored skin, lips, gums, and fingernail beds due to lack of oxygen. This condition may be present in patients with fluid overload that have no yet reached congestive heart failure stage. This condition also accompanies methemoglobinemia, caused by exposure to dialysate water contaminated with nitrates.

CYANOTIC - The nature of an affected area to turn blue due to the lack of oxygen.

CYTOLOGY - The science that deals with the formation, the structure, and the function of cells.

DALTON - The molecular weight or average weight of a molecule (solute) that is measured in Daltons. (Dialyzers can be selected to remove solutes ranging in size from 3,000 Daltons to more than 15,000 daltons).

DEHYDRATION - Dehydration is a condition that occurs when the body does not have enough water. If dehydration occurs, due to repeated diarrhea, vomiting, excess sweating or excess fluid removal during dialysis, the patient may have low blood pressure, sunken eyes, listlessness (lack of interest in surroundings), and poor skin tugor (tone). (*See also: Hypotension*).

DEIONIZER - A deionizer is a component of a water treatment system that uses beds of resin beads to remove unwanted ions from water. The dionizer may have one bed to remove cations and a second bed of anions, and a third; mixed bed to remove all ions. The unwanted ions are exchanged for hydrogen (H+) and hydroxide (OH-) ions from water (H2O). (*See also: Cation, Ion*).

DELIVERY SYSTEM - Mechanism for producing properly mixed dialyzing solution from dialysis concentrate and treated water and delivering it to the artificial kidney at a temperature of 37 ° C. (*See also Hemodialysis Delivery System*).

DIABETES MELLITUS - A chronic disorder of carbohydrate metabolism, characterized by hyperglycemia and glycosuria and resulting from inadequate production or utilization of insulin. Persons fulfilling these conditions are not a homogenous group. Diabetes Mellitus is classified according to two syndromes: Type I, or insulin-dependent diabetes mellitus (IDDM) and type II, or non-insulin dependent diabetes mellitus (NIDDM).

DIABETIC NEPHROPATHY - Diabetic Nephropathy is kidney disease that occurs as a result of diabetes. Diabetes, a failure of the body to utilize glucose (sugar), is the leading cause of renal failure in the U.S. Diabetes also causes damage to the small arteries in the body, which supply blood to the eyes, kidneys, nervous system, and gastrointestinal system.

DIALYSATE - Dialysate is a mixture of treated water and carefully measured chemical that is used to clean the patient's blood during dialysis. Substance such as sodium, calcium, magnesium, chloride, potassium, glucose, and bicarbonate are usually present in the dialysate, in concentrations, similar to normal blood. These concentrations must be very precise, and the dialysate must be mixed properly, or patients can be harmed. In hemodialysis, a semi permeable membrane separates blood and dialysate. Wastes in the blood diffuse across the membrane and into the dialysate, while needed substances diffuse into the blood from the dialysate. In peritoneal dialysis, blood and dialysate are separated by the peritoneum, which acts like a semipermeable membrane. (*See also: Hemodialysis, Osmosis, And Semipermeable Membrane*).

DIALYSATE DELIVERY SYSTEM - See Hemodialysis Delivery System.

DIALYSATE PATH - Conduit through which the dialyzing solution and dialysate pass.

DIALYSIS - Dialysis is a process of removing wastes and excess fluid from the body that damaged kidneys can no longer remove. To maximize the patient's health, the physician will usually prescribe a special renal diet, medications, and other treatments that serve as a supplement to dialysis therapy. Dialysis may be performed using an artificial kidney or dialyzer (hemodialysis) or the patient's own peritoneum (peritoneal dialysis). A dialyzer (containing a semipermeable membrane), dialysate and delivery system are needed to perform hemodialysis. (*See also: Dialysate, Hemodialysis, Hemodialysis Delivery System, Peritoneal Dialysis, and Semipermeable Membrane*).

DIALYSIS ACIDOSIS - Metabolic acidosis due to prolonged hemodialysis in which the pH of the dialysis bath has been inadvertently reduced by the action of contaminating bacteria.

DIALYSIS CHAIN - A dialysis chain is a corporation that owns many facilities, often in different parts of the country. Each year, the larger chains grow in size independent, hospital-based, and smaller chains are incorporated into the larger chains.

DIALYSIS DEMENTIA - See Encephalopathy.

DIALYSIS DISEQUILIBRIUM SYNDROME - Dialysis disequilibrium syndrome is a condition in which rapid or drastic changes in the patient's extracellular fluid affect the brain. Urea transfers more slowly from the brain tissue to the blood, so fluid is drawn into the brain, causing swelling. Dialysis disequilibrium syndrome occurs most often in acute renal failure, or when BUN values are very high. (*See also: Blood Urea Nitrogen*).

DIALYSIS PRINCIPLES - Dialysis principles are basic scientific processes that make dialysis possible: flow, pressure, resistance, solute transfer (primarily by diffusion), filtration, diffusion and osmosis. The dialysis principles help us to understand what happens within the body, the dialyzer, and the delivery system during the process of dialysis therapy. (*See also: Filtration, Flow, Osmosis, Pressure, and Resistance*).

DIALYZER - The dialyzer, or hemodialyzer (also known as the artificial kidney), is a manufactured semipermeable membrane encased in plastic support structure. Dialyzers are used in hemodialysis to remove wastes and fluid from the blood of patients with kidney failure. The semipermeable membrane keeps blood and dialysate separate but allows an exchange of certain solutes and fluids to occur. (*See also: Hollow Fiber Dialyzer, Semipermeable Membrane*).

DIALYZER REPROCESSING - See reprocessing, reuse.

DIALYZING SOLUTION - A properly mixed isotonic solution that is on the opposite site of the membrane from blood in the dialyzer. It is used to set up a concentration gradient within the artificial kidney.

DIASTOLIC - Diastolic pressure is the least pressure of blood against the arteries when the heart is at rest (or between beats). It is the bottom number of a blood pressure reading. (*See also: Systolic*).

DIFFUSION - Diffusion is a scientific principle meaning: dissolved solutes/particles will move form an area of greater concentration to an area of lesser concentration across a semipermeable membrane until the concentration of solutes/particles are equal on both sides of the membrane. In dialysis, diffusion works to remove excess solutes/particles (i.e. waste products) from the blood. Because dialysate is formulated with no wastes (BUN and creatinine), wastes in the blood diffuse across the membrane into the dialysate. The speed of diffusion depends on many factors, such as concentration difference between fluids (concentration gradient), the temperature of dialysate, the size of pores in the semipermeable membrane, and the size of particles. Diffusion is also called conductive solute transport.

DISEQUILIBRIUM SYNDROME - See Dialysis Disequilibrium Syndrome.

DISINFECTION - The process of disinfecting a surface or material with a disinfectant to inhibit the growth of harmful microbes.

DISINFECTANT - A disinfectant is a substance used to destroy or inhibit the growth of microbes. Disinfectant require time to act, and must remain moist and in contact with a surface to be effective. Commonly used for dialysis equipment include formaldehyde, bleach, and gluteraldehye. Commonly used disinfectants for dialyzer reprocessing equipment include formaldehyde, renalin, gluteraldehyde, citric acid, and amuchina. Other uses for disinfectants in dialysis includes cleaning ports on components of the water treatment system before taking a water sample, and wiping off surfaces in the dialysis facilities. (Hibicleans, and Betadine are favorites.)

DISTAL - Distal means far. In anatomy, distal is far from the center of the body. The hands and feet are distal extremities.

DISTAL CONVOLUTED TUBULE - The distal convoluted tubule is located in the kidney, which lies between the Loop of Henle and the collecting duct. (*See also: Ilius*).

DIURESIS - Increased output of urine.

DIURETIC - A diuretic is a medication that increases the amount of urine produced. The use of certain diuretics can lead to hypokalemia because they promote the loss of potassium in urine. Diuretics are used for patient's pre-ESRD, or prior to starting dialysis. (*See also: Hypokalemia*).

DOCUMENTATION - Documentation is a recording of information regarding the patient's care into the permanent medical record or chart. Documentation is important to track the patient's progress, provide a means to follow up each patient's response to treatment, and ensure continuity of care. A patient's medical record provides legal evidence of the care the patient received. Units have specific policies and procedures for documenting patient care.

DORSAL CAVITY - The body cavity that is located toward the back (posterior) of the body, it is divided into the cranial cavity which contains the brain and the vertebral cavity, which contains the spinal cord.

DRIP CHAMBER / BUBBLE TRAP - An arterial or venous drip chamber reflects arterial or venous pressure in the extracorporeal circuit, using a monitoring line. A bubble trap inside the drip chamber collects any air that may have accidentally entered the blood tubing.

DRY ULTRAFILTRATION - See isolated ultrafiltration (DUF, IUF, PUF).

DRY WEIGHT - A person with renal failure is said to be at a "dry weight" if there are no signs of fluid overload or dehydration, respiration is normal—with out evidence of fluid in the lungs—and the blood pressure is normal for the patient, neither too high nor too low. "Target weight" is the goal weight for a particular dialysis treatment, and is usually determined by the dry weight.

DWELL TIME - In hemodialysis, dwell time is the length of time a disinfectant needs to stay in a dialyzer long enough to ensure proper disinfection during reprocessing. Also for hemodialysis delivery system disinfection, if a chemical disinfectant is used, it must dwell in the delivery system fluid pathways long enough to kill bacteria, and then thoroughly rinse. In peritoneal dialysis, dwell time is the length of time dialysate remains inside the patient's abdomen before it is drained out and replaced with fresh dialysate. (*See also: Reprocessing*).

DYSPNEA - Dyspnea mean trouble breathing, or shortness of breath. Dyspnea can be a symptom of anemia, fluid overload, lung or heart problems, or other dialysis complications such as air embolism (air entering the bloodstream). (*See also: Air Embolism, Anemia, Pulmonary Edema, and Uremia*).

ECCHYMOSIS - An ecchymosis is a bruise or bleeding under the skin, causing skin discoloration. In dialysis patients, ecchymosis can be a sign that too much heparin has been administered or that inadequate pressure was placed on the needle site after the needles were removed.

EDEMA - Edema is water retention/swelling in the body tissues that occurs as a result of fluid overload or other conditions. The swelling may be observed in the patient's eyelids, ankles, feet, hands, abdomen, or lower back area. "Pitting" edema is when a finger is pushed against the skin of the ankles and leaving a dent. This condition should be reported to a nurse (If it is new for that patient). (*See also: Dry weight, Pulmonary Edema*).

EFFERENT ARTERIOLE - A small artery that carries blood away from the glomeruli of the kidney.

ELECTROLYTE - An electrolyte is a compound (such as sodium, potassium, and calcium) that breaks apart into ions (electrically charged particles) when dissolved in water. Electrolytes transport electrical impulses along the nerves to the muscles, including the heart. In the body, healthy kidneys maintain electrolyte balance. Electrolytes are added to the dialysate in carefully controlled amounts. Also called <u>ions</u> and can be positive or negative charged particles.

EMBOLUS – A mass of undissolved matter present in a blood vessel, which may be solid, liquid or gaseous. Emboli can cause occlusion or blockage of the vessel. (*See also: Air Embolism*).

EMPTY BED CONTACT TIME - Empty bed contact time is the time period during which the feed water must remain in contact with the charcoal bed in a carbon tank during water treatment. Feed water must remain in contact with the charcoal long enough to allow adequate removal of chlorine and chloramines. (*See also: Carbon Tank, Chloramines, and Feed Water*).

ENCEPHALOPATHY - Encephalopathy is a defect in the function of brain tissues that can be fatal. The symptoms include confusion, short-term memory problems, personality changes, speech problems, muscle spasms, hallucinations, seizure and intellectual impairment. One cause of encephalopathy is chronic exposure to high levels of aluminum in dialysis water. Sources of aluminum include dialysate water, antacids, laxatives, and cookware.

ENDOCARDIUM - Serous lining membrane of inner surface and cavities of the heart. It is continuous with the intimae or the interior coat of arteries.

ENDOCRINE FUNCTION - Endocrine function, the production of hormones, is one of the tasks of healthy kidneys. Kidneys manufacture hormones that adjust blood pressure (angiotensin) and stimulate red blood cells formation (erythropoietin). Healthy kidneys also convert vitamin D into an activated for that the body can use to absorb calcium to maintain healthy bones (Calcitriol). (*See also: Hormones*).

ENDOTOXIN - Endotoxins (lippopolysaccharide) is a toxic component that forms part of the cell walls of bacteria. Licing bacteria can shed endotoxin, and endotoxins are also released when bacteria die and decompose. Because endotoxins are <u>not alive</u>, disinfectants cannot kill it. However, if endotoxin is allowed to enter the patient's body, it can cause pyrogenic (fever) reactions. Endotoxin is a concern in water treatment and dialyzer reprocessing; numbers are decreased by reducing the numbers of bacteria in the water or by using an ultrafilter to remove endotoxin. (*See also: Pyrogenic Reaction, Ultrafilter*).

END-STAGE RENAL DISEASE (ESRD) - ESRD is a legal term for complete and irreversible loss of kidney function, the last stage of chronic renal failure, when renal replacement therapy must be started if the patient is to live. Patients are generally considered to have ESRD when the glomerular filtration rate has dropped to about 10% of normal. (5 to 10 ml/min). (*See also: Chronic Renal Failure, Glomerular Filtration Rate*).

EPICARDIUM - The inner visceral layer of the pericardium, which forms a serous membrane, forming the outermost layer of the wall of the heart.

EPOGEN (EPOETIN ALFA) - Epogen is a recombinant (cloned) form of erythropoietin, a hormone that stimulates the bone morrow to form red blood cells. EPOGEN injected intravenously (into a vein) or subcutaneously (into the tissue beneath the skin), is used to treat anemia of chronic renal failure, eliminating the need for most blood transfusions in dialysis patients and improving their quality of life. Common side effects include hypertension and flu-like symptoms. (*See also: Anemia, Erythropoietin, and Recombinant*).

EQUILIBRIUM - Equilibrium is the state of balance. Diffusion (the movement of solutes) occurs until there is an equal concentration on both sides of a semipermeable membrane-until equilibrium has been reached. (*See also: Diffusion, Osmosis, and Semipermeable Membrane*).

ERYTHROCYTE - A mature red blood cell or corpuscle. The body of the cell consists of a sponge-like stroma containing a respiratory pigment, hemoglobin, enclosed in a cell membrane of proteins in combination with lipoid substances.

ERYTHROPOIETIN (EPO) - Erythropoietin is a hormone produced by healthy kidneys that stimulates bone marrow to produce red blood cells. Anemia caused by using EPOGEN can now treat a shortage of erythropoietin in dialysis patients. Epotin Alfa is a synthetic form of erythropoietin. (*See also: Anemia*).

ESRD - See End Stage Renal Disease.

ESRD NETWORKS - The ESRD networks were established by the U.S government in 1978 to oversee dialysis facilities and ensure that patients receive high quality care. The networks collect data, implement quality improvement, encourage rehabilitation, establish a grievance procedure for patients, and provide resource materials to ESRD for staff and patients.

EHTYLENE OXIDE (ETO) - ETO is a gas used by some manufacturers to sterilize new dialyzers. Patients who are hypersensitive to ETO may suffer the effects of first use syndrome if a new dialyzer that has been sterilized with ETO is not properly rinsed. (ETO is ethylene oxide). (*See also: First Use Syndrome, Hypersensitivity*).

EXCRETORY FUNCTION -To excrete means to eliminate from the body. An important excretory function of healthy kidneys it is to rid the body of wastes and excess fluid by producing urine. Urine contains excess body water and a high concentration of waste products.

EXSANGUINATION - Exsanguination is the severe loss of blood that may be life threatening. Common preventable causes of exsanguinations include needle dislodgment, bloodline separation, access rupture, or cracked dialyzer casing.

EXTRACELLULAR - Extracellular means outside the cells or surrounding the tissue and also includes the interstitial and intravascular compartments. Extracellular fluid makes up about 1/3 of all the fluid in the body at any given time. Of this fluid about 2/3 is found between organ tissues (interstitial), and the rest is the vascular space (blood vessels), to be removed by dialysis. The sodium level in the dialysate helps ensure the movement of fluid from one fluid compartment to the other.

EXTRACELLULAR FLUID - Tissue fluid or fluid occupying spaces between the spaces of cells.

EXTRACORPOREAL - Extracorporeal means outside of the body. Hemodialysis is extracorporeal therapy, because it takes place outside the body.

EXTRACORPOREAL CIRCUIT - The extracorporeal circuit is an extension of the patient's blood vessels outside of the body. The circuit carries the patient's blood from the access to the dialyzer, and back to the patient. Components of the extracorporeal circuit include the arterial bloodline, dialyzer, venous bloodline, and extracorporeal circuit monitors. (*See also: Blood Tubing, Dialyzer*).

EXTRACORPOREAL CIRCUIT MONITORS - The extra corporeal circuit monitors include blood flow monitor, arterial or venous pressure monitors (measured at the drip chambers), an air detector, and a blood leak detector. These monitors shut off the blood pump and clamp the venous bloodline when the present limits are exceeded on the arterial and venous bloodline, or when blood is detected in the spent dialysate by the blood leak detector. (*See also: Air Detector, Arterial Pressure, Blood Leak Detector, and Venous Pressure*).

EXTRACORPOREAL SYSTEM - The venous and arterial bloodlines that includes the dialyzer for the hemodialysis machine. (*See also: Extracorporeal Circuit*).

EXTRASKELETAL CALCIFICATION - Extraskeletal calcification is the depositing of crystals of calcium phosphate in the patient's blood vessels or soft tissues. The condition can potentially cause gangrene. Hypercalcemia with hyperphosphatemia can cause extraskeletal calcification. Mottled, painful, purplish skin is a symptom of extraskeletal calcification that should be reported immediately to the nurse or nephrologist. (*See also: Hypercalcemia, Hyperphosphatemia*).

FEED WATER - Feed water is untreated tap water before it passes through a water treatment system. Feed water must pass through the various components of a water treatment system before being used for dialysis.

FEMORAL CATHETER - A femoral catheter is a temporary vascular access placed in the femoral vein in the groin. The femoral vein is easy to reach and preserves blood vessels in the upper body for permanent vascular access. However, the site is very prone to infection and limits the patient's mobility. Therefore, it is typically used for critically ill or bedridden patients.

FEMORAL VEIN - A continuation of the popliteal vein upward toward the external iliac vein.

FERRITIN - Ferritin is an iron storage protein complex that occurs in body tissues and is measured with a blood test. Adequate ferritin stores are necessary to help ensure that EPOGEN can be effectively utilized to stimulate red blood cell production.

FIBER BUNDLE VOLUME (FBV) - Fiber bundle volume, also called total cell volume (TCV), is a measure of the volume of fluid that the hollow fibers in a dialyzer can hold. Fiber bundle volume is measured before a dialyzer is used for the first time and again after each reprocessing, because reprocessing a dialyzer can alter the FBV. (*See also: Reprocessing*).

FIBRIN - A whitish filamentous protein formed by the action of thrombin or fibrogen. The fibrin is deposited, as fine interlacing filaments is which are entangled red and white blood cells and platelets, the whole forming a coagulum or clot.

FIBRIN SHEATH - A fibrin sheath is a collection of blood clotting fibers on the outside of a catheter lumen. The fibers can form a cap that blocks the end of a catheter and reduces blood flow. (*See also: Catheter, Lumen*).

FIBROSIS - Fibrosis is the overgrowth of scar tissue. Fibrosis can develop in a fistula as a result of repeated needle punctures for dialysis. The scar tissue builds up, gradually narrowing the lumen of the vessel and reducing the blood flow. (*See also: Arterio Venous Fistula, Lumen*).

FILTERS - Filters are devices that remove particles, solutes, and other substances of a given size by passing them through holes of various sizes. Sediment filters are components of dialysis water treatment systems that trap undissolved particles such as sand and mud before they can reach the reverse osmosis membrane and damage it. Depth filters are a type of sediment filter that may contain one or more layers of fibrous material or mesh, each layer finer than the one before, to trap smaller and smaller particles. These filters can remove nearly all-floating particles from the feed water.

FILTRATION - Filtration is the process of passing fluid through a filter. In dialysis, filtration forces fluid out of the patient's blood and across the dialyzer membrane by using pressure.

FIRST USE SYNDROME - First use syndrome is a group of symptoms that may occur shortly after the beginning of a dialysis treatment with a new dialyzer. Symptoms may include nervousness, chest pain, back pain, palpitations, (skipped or missed heartbeats) or itching. First use syndrome may be caused by exposure to ethylene oxide gas or manufacturing residues remaining in the dialyzer after production. Pre-processing a dialyzer may reduce the incidence of first use syndrome by removing ethylene oxide and manufacturing residues called plasticizers. A coating of blood protein remaining in the dialyzer after dialysis also makes a reprocessed dialyzer more biocompatible—unless the coating is removed by bleach during reprocessing. (*See also: Biocompatible, Cellulose, Ethylene Oxide, and Reprocessing*).

FISTULA - Unnatural opening or passage. In dialysis, the result of anastamosis of an artery to a vein to allow access to the blood stream for hemodialysis. *(See also Arteriovenous Fistula).*

FLOCCULANT - A flocculant is a chemical added to a municipal water supply to make the water clearer. Alum is one substance that may be used a flocculant. (*See also: Alum*).

FLOW - Flow is a stream. Blood flow to each organ in the body is determined by the amount and pressure of blood delivered by the heart, and the resistance of the blood meets in the blood vessels. The setting of the blood pump, resistance in the extracorporeal circuit, and capacity of the vascular access determine blood flow in the extracorporeal circuit.

FLUID DYNAMICS – A description of how two fluids, blood and dialysate, are pumped through tubing systems. (Within the dialyzer, blood and dialysate are separated from each other by a semipermeable membrane).

FLUID MOVEMENT - See osmosis.

FLUSH - See priming.

FOOD AND DRUG ADMINISTRATION (FDA) - The FDA is a federal office that regulates the release and marketing of medications and medical devices, including dialyzers and devices used for reprocessing.

FORMALDEHYDE - Formaldehyde is a poisonous, colorless, foul-smelling gas. In its liquid form (37% gas in water) it is called aqueous formaldehyde or Formalin, and it is an effective germicide used for disinfecting dialysate delivery systems, or for reprocessing dialyzers. The liquid form is volatile, changing readily into vapor that can penetrate and disinfect even small spaces. Formaldehyde is a suspected cancer-causing agent; facilities must follow OSHA safety procedures to prevent injury to patients or staff.

FORMALIN - Formalin is a trademark name for a 37% solution of formaldehyde.

FREE CHLORINE - Free chlorine is chlorine that is not chemically bound to other substances. (*See also: Chloramines*).

FRONTAL PLANE - A plane parallel with the long axis of the body and at right angles to the median sagittal plane. A plane that divides the body into anterior and posterior sections.

FUNCTIONAL STATUS - Functional status is an individual's ability to perform usual activities, such as walking, cooking, dressing, toileting, working, attending school, etc.

GASTROPARESIS – Delayed emptying of food from the stomach into the small bowel. Gastroparesis may be a chronic complication of diseases marked by autonomic failure such as diabetes mellitus, chronic renal failure and amyloidosis.

GERMICIDE - A germicide is a germ-killing solution. Germicides are used in reprocessing dialyzers. (*See also: Dialyzer, Formalin, Reprocessing, and Solution*).

GLANDS - A secretory organ or structure. A cell group or a group of cells that can manufacture a secretion discharged and used in some other part of the body.

GLOMERULAR FILTRATE - Glomerular filtrate is a watery fluid left when the blood is filtered by healthy kidneys. It is the protein free plasma from which urine is formed. Low molecular weight substances (small waste particles and water) pass through tiny pores in the glomeruli and into Bowman's space. A healthy adult produces about 180 liters of glomerular filtrate per day. (*See also: Glomerulus*).

GLOMERULAR FILTRATION - The process of fluid passing from the blood through the capillary walls of the glomeruli of the kidney to be filtered.

GLOMERULAR FILTRATION RATE (GFR) - The GFR is the volume of blood filtered by the glomerulus each minute, in ml/min. A normal GRF is about 120 to 130 ml/min. People with kidney failure have GFR's that are below normal.

GLOMERULONEPHRITIS - Glomerulonephritis is an inflammation that damages the glomeruli of the kidneys. Hypertension often accompanies glomerulonephritis. Glomerulonephritis can be slow and progressive or rapid in onset, and sometimes occurs as an immune response to a streptococcal infection. (The incidence of glomerulonephritis has decreased significantly over the past 20 years as a result of earlier treatment of streptococcal infection).

GLOMERULUS - The glomerulus is a tangled ball of capillaries that are a part of a kidney nephron. Water and small molecular weight particles are forced through filtration silts in each glomerulus by the pressure of the beating heart. The resulting solution is called glomerular filtrate.

GRADIENT - A gradient is a difference. A concentration gradient is a difference in the concentration of solutes of two different fluids, separated by a semipermeable membrane. In dialysis the fluids are blood and dialysate separated by a dialyzer membrane in hemodialysis or by the peritoneum in the peritoneal dialysis.

GRAFT - To graft is to join one thing surgically to another. In hemodialysis, a graft is a piece of artificial vessel that can be used to create an access. One end of the graft is connected to the patient's artery, the other to the vein.

GRAM-NEGATIVE - Gram-negative bacteria are a class of bacteria that turn pink in a standard laboratory Gram's stain. They have adapted especially to survive in water. These bacteria form an electrically charged bio-film (slime) that allows them to cling to surfaces, such as dialysate containers or hoses. The biofilm protects the bacteria from disinfectants, making them difficult to remove. For example Acromobacter is a Gram-negative bacteria that can contaminate in the dialysis water supply or the dialysate. Acinetobacter, Aeromonas, Alcaligenes, Flavobacterium, Moraxella, Pseudomonas, and Serratia are other types of Gram-Negative bacteria.

GRAM-POSITIVE BACTERIA - Gram-positive bacteria turn blue to black in a standard laboratory Gram's stain. Staphylococci are gram-positive bacteria that cause most access infections.

GUAIAC CARDS - Guaiac Cards are used to test for hidden (occult) blood in stool. A developing solution is dipped onto a smear of stool on a Guaiac card. If the stain turns blue, blood is present. Guiac cards may be used with patients with low hematocrit or hemoglobin levels to determine if gastrointestinal bleeding is occurring. (*See also: Anemia*).

HARD WATER - The total concentration of calcium and magnesium in water.

HEADERS - A plastic cap covering the ends of the hollow fibers enclosed in the plastic casing (dialyzer).

HEALTH CARE FINANCING ADMINISTRATION (HCFA) - HCFA is a federal agency that oversees Medicare and other health related agencies. Dialyzer reprocessing and the related health standards and conditions of reprocessing are also regulated by HCFA.

HEAT DISINFECTION - An alternative to chemical disinfectants used to reprocess certain types of dialyzer and to disinfect dialysis equipment (that is equipped with this feature). Heat disinfection prevents patient and staff exposure to chemicals. Cellulose-based dialyzer membranes degrade during heat disinfection, and therefore cannot be disinfected using heat.

HEMASTIX - A reagent strip that reacts to the presence of blood. When the blood leak detector indicates the presence of blood in the used dialysate and the blood is not visible, a Hemastix should be used to determine the presence and the extent of the leak. (*See also: Blood Leak Detector, Dialysate*).

HEMATOCRIT - A measure of red blood cells in the blood, stated as a percentage of red blood cells per total blood volume. Routinely checking hematocrit levels allows clinicians to assess anemia, follow the patient's response to EPOGEN, and alert the staff to any chronic loss of blood. NKF-DOQI guidelines recommend a target hematocrit level for dialysis patients of 33% to 36%. (*See also: Anemia, EPOGEN, and Hemoglobin*).

HEMATOMA - A painful, hard, discolored (black-and-blue) collection of blood under the skin, caused by blood escaping from a vessel into surrounding tissue. Hematomas can form during or after placement of dialysis needles and when needles are removed.

HEMOCONCENTRATION - The dehydration of the blood, which can occur in the extracorporeal circuit if ultrafiltration continues after the blood pump is turned off, or if recirculation within the access is occurring. Hemoconcentration can lead to blood clotting.

HEMODIALYSIS - A process that cleans the blood of waste products by passing the blood through an artificial kidney, or dialyzer. Blood and dialysate are passed through the membrane, and into the dialysate according to the principles of diffusion and osmosis. Hemodialysis is the most commonly chosen treatment modality for patients with end-stage renal disease.

HEMODIALYSIS ADEQUACY - A measure of the dose of dialysis a patient receives to be sure enough dialysis is given to allow the patient to feel well and have a good quality of life. The first clinical practice guidelines, developed by the Renal Physicians Association (RPA).

HEMODIALYSIS DELIVERY SYSTEM - A machine that consists of a blood pump, dialysis solution, dialysate, delivery system, and appropriate safety monitors. The blood pump moves blood from the patient's access side through the dialyzer and back to the patient. The machine prepares dialysate by mixing specially treated water with the dialysate concentrate. The delivery system also controls and monitors dialysate conductivity, temperature, flow rate, and pressure. (*See also: Extracorporeal Circuit*).

HEMODIALYZER - See dialyzer.

HEMOGLOBIN - Hemoglobin is the oxygen-carrying pigment of red blood cells. Measuring hemoglobin levels is a means of diagnosing anemia. Routinely checking hemoglobin levels allows clinicians to follow the patient's response to EPOGEN and alerts the staff to any chronic blood loss. NKF-DOQI guidelines recommend a target hemoglobin range of between 11 and 12 g/dl. The EPOGEN package insert recommends a target hemoglobin range of 10 to 12 g/dl. (*See also: Anemia, EPOGEN*).

HEMOLYSIS - The destruction of red blood cells by bursting, a life-threatening condition that requires immediate attention from a physician. Hemolysis may be caused by hyponatremia (low blood sodium); overheated dialysate; too diluted (hypotonic) dialysate; chloramines, copper, or nitrates in the dialysate water; formaldehyde or bleach in the dialysate; low-conductivity (too much water and not enough concentrate); too high prepump arterial pressure; incompatible blood transfusions; occlusion or kinking of blood tubing; some medications; and certain diseases.

HEMOLYTIC ANEMIA - Anemia resulting from hemolysis of red blood cells acquired from the effects of toxic agents.

HEMOTHORAX - A collection of blood in the chest that prevents the lungs from fully expanding, causing difficulty breathing. Hemothorax can occur if a blood vessel is accidentally punctured during placement of a dialysis catheter.

HEPARIN - An anticoagulant or an anticlotting medication, given during dialysis to allow blood to flow freely through the extracorporeal circuit.

HEPARIN INFUSION LINE - The heparin line is a very small in diameter tube that extends out of the blood tubing that allows the administration of heparin during dialysis. The heparin infusion line is normally located on the arterial blood-tubing segment just before the dialyzer.

HEPARIN PUMP - A heparin fusion pump consists of a syringe holder, a piston, and an electric motor, and is used to continuously to deliver precise amounts of heparin during dialysis. The heparin pump is connected to the heparin infusion line, which is part of the extracorporeal blood tubing. Most dialysis machines produced today include a heparin delivery system, although stand-alone heparin pumps are still in use in some settings.

HEPATITIS - Hepatitis is an inflammation of the liver caused by a virus that can be found in several forms, including hepatitis viruses A, B (HBV) or C (HCV). Because hepatitis B and C are spread through contact with infected blood or other body fluid, they are a concern for hemodialysis patients and staff. Hepatitis virus infections can cause long-term and permanent liver damage or death. Vaccination against the hepatitis B virus should be offered to all dialysis staff members and patients. Standard precautions should be followed to prevent the spread of hepatitis, as well as other infections.

HEPATORENAL SYNDROME - Condition in which the patient exhibits both kidney and liver failure.

HIGH-EFFICIENCY DIALYSIS - High efficiency dialysis uses dialyzers that are capable of removing more small solutes (i.e., urea) than conventional membranes. Blood flow rates ranging from 300 to 500 ml/min are usually used, as well as having UF control when dialysis is done with a dialyzer's KUF above 8. *(See also: Coefficient of Ultrafiltration)*.

HIGH-EFFICIENCY DIALYZER – Dialyzers with medium to large surface areas (1.3 – 2.2 square meters), medium KUFs (8 – 12 ml/mmHg/hr) and low molecular weight cutoffs (3,000 Daltons). These dialyzers can be made of cellulose or synthetic material and must be used with ultrafiltration control machines. (*See also: High-efficiency dialysis*).

HIGH-FLUX DIALYSIS - High-flux dialysis uses a membrane permeable to a broad range of molecular weight solutes, including higher molecular weight solutes. Kuf's for high-flux dialysis are higher than 8, making ultrafiltration control mandatory. High-flux dialyzers have the ability to remove larger amounts of fluid as well as large substances such as beta-2-microglobulin or B_2M.

HIGH-FLUX DIALYZER – Dialyzers with medium too large surface areas (up to 2.0 square meters), high KUFs (12 – 60+ ml/mmHg/hr) and high molecular weight cutoffs (15,000 Daltons). These dialyzers are made of synthetic material and tend to be more biocompatible. These dialyzers must, also, be used with ultrafiltration control machines. (*See also: High-flux dialysis*).

HIGH-OUTPUT CARDIAC FAILURE – Condition that occurs when the patient's heart grows larger, but still cannot work hard enough to pump out the extra blood sent to the heart by placement of an AV fistula or graft. (*See also: Cardiac Output*).

HISTOLOGY - The study of microscopic structure of tissue.

HOLOW FIBER – Dialyzer membrane material (cellulose or synthetic) formed into thin tubes enclosed in a plastic case that holds the dialyzer together and provides pathways for blood and dialysate to flow in and out of the dialyzer.

HOLLOW FIBER DIALYZER - The hollow fiber dialyzer contains thousands of tiny hollow fibers (semipermeable membranes), held in place at each end by clay-like potting material. The hollow fiber and potting material are encased in a hard plastic cylinder. During dialysis the blood flows through the hollow tubes, and dialysate is circulated around them. The hollow fiber dialyzer allows for well-controlled and predictable diffusion and ultrafiltration, and is currently the only type of dialyzer available in the U.S. (*See also: Dialyzer, Diffusion, and Ultrafiltration*).

HOMEOSTASIS - The relatively constant balance naturally maintained in the internal environment of the body. Healthy kidneys help maintain fluid balance, acid/base balance, hormonal balance, and electrolyte balance, all-important component of homeostasis.

HORMONES - Chemical substances produced on one organ or gland of the body that act on a different organ. Healthy kidneys produce a hormone (erythropoietin) that causes red blood cells to be manufactured by the bone marrow, and other hormones that maintain blood pressure and regulate calcium metabolism.

HUMAN IMMUNODEFICIENCY VIRUS (HIV) - A virus that disables the body's immune system by destroying white blood cells that fight disease (T-lymphocytes). HIV is transmitted through blood, semen, vaginal secretions, peritoneal fluids, and breast milk, Over time, people infected with HIV can develop immunodeficiency syndrome (AIDS). Damage to the immune system caused by AIDS leaves the body vulnerable to infections and cancers the usually do not occur in people with healthy immune systems. While new treatments are available, prevention is the best approach. Follow standard precautions to prevent the spread of HIV in the dialysis unit. (*See also: Infection Control, Opportunistic Illness, and Standard Precautions*).

HYDRAULIC PRESSURE - Water pressure created naturally (such as from gravity) or artificially (such as from a pump). Hydraulic pressure is one factor that affects the amount of water that will be removed from the patient during dialysis.

HYDROSTATIC PRESSURE - Pressure produced by the height of a column of fluid.

HYPER - The prefix hyper means beyond, above, more, or too much. For example, hyperactivity is an above normal activity level.

HYPERCALCEMIA – Means too much calcium (an electrolyte) in the blood. Patient symptoms of hypercalcemia can include muscle weakness, fatigue, constipation, loss of appetite, abdominal cramps, nausea, vomiting, and coma. (*See also: Electrolyte*).

HYPERKALEMIA - Means too much potassium (an electrolyte) in the blood. Hyperkalemia causes symptoms of muscle weakness, and can lead to cardiac arrhythmias, cardiac arrest, or death. Hyperkalemia can occur if the dialysis patient eats too man high potassium foods; if there is tissue breakdown due to surgery, bleeding, hemolysis, or fever; or if dialysate with too much potassium is used. These conditions cause potassium to be released from cells into the bloodstream. (*See also: Electrolyte*).

HYPERMAGNESEMIA - Means too much magnesium (an electrolyte) in the blood. Magnesium is needed for muscle and nerve functioning. Symptoms of hypermagnesmia include impaired nerve transmission, hypotension, respiratory depression, and sleepiness. Severe hypermagnesmia can cause cardiac arrest. (*See also: Electrolyte*).

HYPERNATREMIA - Means too much sodium (an electrolyte) in the blood. Excess sodium in the blood causes water to move out of the cells—including red blood cells – and into the extracellular space. Hypernatremia can cause headaches, hypertension, and crenation, a shrinkage of red blood cells that can be fatal. (*See also: Electrolyte*).

HYPERPARATHYROID BONE DISEASE – A bone disease or condition resulting from over activity of the parathyroid glands causing excessive levels of parathyroid hormone (PTH) in the body with resulting disturbances in calcium and phosphorus metabolism. It is characterized by decalcification of the bone, elevated levels of blood calcium, lowering levels of blood phosphorus, and kidney stones.

HYPERPHOSPHATEMIA - Means too much phosphorus in the blood. Phosphorous is a component of bones, and is also key in energy transfer between cells. When combined with hypercalcemia, hyperphosphatemia can cause crystal deposits in soft tissues, fractures and bone pain. Hyperphosphatemia is usually found in patients who are eating more than the prescribed amount of protein and or dairy products, not taking enough phosphate binders, or not timing the ingestion of phosphate binders to coincide with their meals.

HYPERPLASIA – Is the overgrowth of cells. Clotting that occurs in the middle of a vascular access graft is often caused by clumps of platelets developing on areas of hyperplasia.

HYPERSENSITIVITY - An excessive or abnormal sensitivity or allergy. Hypersensitivity reactions occur most often with cuprophane dialyzer, and can even lead to anaphylaxis in some patients. (*See also: Anaphylactic Reaction*).

HYPERTENSION - Means high blood pressure. In the adult, a condition in which the B/P is higher than 140/90 on three separate readings recorded several weeks apart. Hypertension can be a cause or a result of kidney failure; it is the second most common cause of kidney disease in the U.S. Hypertension can damage the kidneys, heart, blood vessels, and other organs.

HYPO - The prefix "hypo" means below, beneath or too little. For example, hypocalcemia means there is too little calcium in the blood. A hypodermic needle is a needle that is inserted below the skin.

HYPOCALCEMIA - Means not enough calcium (an electrolyte) in the blood). Hypocalcemia can cause tetany—spasms and twitching of the muscles or seizures. Low blood calcium can occur in kidney disease due to the loss of calcitrol production by the failing kidneys. Calcitrol allows the body to absorb calcium from the diet. (*See also: Electrolyte*).

HYPOKALEMIA - Means not enough potassium (an electrolyte) in the blood. This condition is unusual in dialysis patients, but can occur when there is not enough potassium in the diet or dialysate. Hypokalemia can also be caused by a loss of potassium, due to vomiting, diarrhea, use of potassium exchange resins, and use of diuretics that can increase the loss of potassium in the urine. (*See also: Electrolyte*).

HYPONATREMIA - Means not enough sodium (an electrolyte) in the blood. Without enough sodium, water moves out of the extracellular space and into cells, which can cause hypotension, muscle cramps, and hemolysis—destruction of red blood cells. (*See also: Electrolyte*).

HYPOPHOSPHATEMIA - Means not enough phosphorous in the blood. This condition is rare in dialysis patients, because phosphorous is found in most foods. Predisponding factors include poor nutritional intake and excessive intake of phosphate binders. Low levels of phosphorous can indicate malnutrition. Serious consequences of hypophosphatemia include cardiac arrhythmias or muscle weakness.

HYPOTENSION - Blood pressure that is abnormally low. A decrease of the B/P below normal, less than 100/60. In dialysis patients, hypotension occurs most commonly when too much fluid is removed during dialysis, or when patients are overmedicated with antihypertensive drugs. Symptoms of hypotension include feeling of warmth, restlessness, dizziness, nausea, or visual disturbance. The trendelenberg—raising the feet higher than the heart—and volume replacement (i.e., normal saline) help relieve hypotension.

HYPOTONIC DIALYSATE - Hypotonic dialysate is dialysate that is diluted with too much water, which can lead to hemolysis. (*See also: Hemolysis*).

IMMUNOSUPPRESSIVE DRUGS - Drugs used to reduce the severity of immune reactions to such substances as protein.

IN-CENTER HEMODIALYSIS - Treatments are performed in a hospital or freestanding dialysis clinic. In-center dialysis is usually assisted by dialysis staff members, although patients may be able to take their own vital signs, place their own needles, and monitor their own treatments.

INFECTION - A condition produced by invasion of the body with a disease-producing organism (i.e., bacteria).

INFECTION CONTROL - A series of steps taken to prevent the spread of infection. Using aseptic technique for invasive procedures, disinfecting equipment after use, washing hands, and wearing protective equipment are all part of infection control. (*See also: Standard Precautions*).

INFILTRATION - An abnormal leakage of a substance into bodily tissues. In dialysis patients, infiltration of blood into the tissues surrounding the vascular access can occur if the needle punctures the back of the vessel wall. To prevent infiltration, needle insertion must be performed carefully.

INFLAMMATION - Tissue swelling in reaction to injury, infection, or surgery.

INORGANIC- Chemical compounds that do not contain carbon. Non-living bacteria.

INSTILL - To place into or to cause to enter. Heparin is instilled into each lumen of a catheter to prevent clotting in the catheter between dialysis treatments. PD fluid is instilled into the peritoneum for peritoneal dialysis.

INTEGRITY – Unimpaired, undiminished state (Pure state).

INTERDIALYTIC - Means between dialysis treatments. Patients must restrict their fluid intake to prevent interdialytic fluid gain that complicates fluid removal during a single hemodialysis treatment.

INTERMITTENT - Means "periodically" or not "continuously". Heparin can be given intermittently throughout dialysis. (*See also: Heparin*).

INTERNAL JUGULAR CATHETER (IJ) - Temporary or permanent dialysis catheters placed in the internal jugular vein in the neck. This location is less likely to cause central venous stenosis than placement in the subclavian vein. (*See also: Central Venous Stenosis*).

INTERNAL JUGULAR VEIN - Any of the two bilateral veins located in the neck that return blood from the head to the heart. In dialysis these veins are used for placement of temporary or permanent dialysis catheters.

INTERSTITIAL FLUID - Fluid that surrounds the cells, in tissue spaces. Tissue fluid.

INTERSTITIAL SPACE - The space between the cells of an organ or tissue.

INTIMA - The smooth lining of the inner surfaces of arteries and veins. The intima is covered with a thin, fragile layer of cells that allows blood to flow through the vessel easily.

INTRACELLULAR - Means within the cells. Sodium causes fluid to move across cell membranes between the intracellular and extracellular spaces. (*See also: Extracellular*).

INTRACELLULAR FLUID – Fluid within the cell, approximately 2/3 of body water.

INTRADERMAL - Means within the skin. Local anesthetics may be injected intradermally.

INTRAMUSCULAR - Means within the muscle.

INTRAVASCULAR - Means with in blood vessels.

INTRAVENOUS - Intravenous means within the vein. Many medications, including EPOGEN, are injected intravenously.

INVITRO - Invitro is a Latin phrase that means outside the human body and in an artificial environment. Dialyzer clearance is measured invitro by the manufacturer; using non-blood fluids (i.e., saline), so actual dialyzer clearance may vary from the manufactures' specifications.

INVIVO - Invivo is a Latin phrase that means within the plant or animal. Tests performed on a dialyzer while a patient is being treated are considered invivo.

ION – Electrically charged particles; electrolytes. Ions are formed when electrons in the outer shell are either gained or lost. Ions carry a positive charge (cation) or a negative charge (anion).

ION EXCHANGE - A process that occurs inside a deionizer for water treatment. Unwanted ions are traded for hydrogen and hydroxyl ions to create pure water. (*See also: Deionizer*).

IRON DEFICIENCY - A lack of sufficiently available iron in the body to make red blood cells. Without iron, which is needed to synthesize hemoglobin, bone marrow cannot make red blood cells, even if erythropoietin levels are sufficient. Low levels of iron can cause a form of anemia. (*See also: Anemia*).

ISCHEMIA - The lack of sufficient oxygen to the tissues, due to reduced blood flow. The affected tissues may have pain. For example, ischemia of the heart can cause angina pain; ischemia of the hand may include symptoms of hand pain during exercise, a cold, clammy feeling and in extreme cases, painful, non-healing skin ulcers. Limb ischemia can be caused by placement or complications of some vascular accesses, and, in severe cases, can lead to loss of a limb.

ISOLATED ULTRAFILTRATION (IU) - An extracorporeal treatment that removes water, but not solutes, by using the extracorporeal circuit and dialyzer without dialysate. IU is also called dry ultrafiltration, sequential ultrafiltration, or pure ultrafiltration. Isolated ultrafiltration can be performed before, after, or independently of dialysis. The principle advantage of IU is that fluid removal is better tolerated that with conventional hemodialysis.

ISOTONIC - Having the same concentration or the same osmotic pressure.

KIDNEY - Paired organs, purple brown in color, situated at the back of the abdominal cavity, one on each side of the spinal column. Their function is to excrete the urine and to help regulate the water, electrolyte, and acid based content of the blood.

KIDNEY TRANSPLANT - A replacement of a diseased kidney with a healthy kidney from a donor. Only one healthy kidney is needed to live. It is possible to receive a donor kidney from a relative, spouse or friend, or a cadaver (deceased). Blood type and other tissue factors are used to "match" a recipient after a medical work-up has been done.

Kt/V – Formula used to determine the actual delivered dose of dialysis. (*See also: Urea Kinetic Modeling, Natural Logarithm*).

KUF – Means the manufacturer's specified ultrafiltration coefficient. The KUF is the amount of fluid removed by the dialyzer in one hour at a given pressure; stated as ml/mmHg/hr. (*See also: Coefficient of Ultrafiltration*).

LABEL (on a REUSE DIALYZER) - The label consists of the name of the patient, the number of times the dialyzer has been reprocessed, the date and time of the last reprocess, the original residual, the total cell or fiber bundle volume, the signature of the person who performed the reprocessing, and the initials of the tech that puts the patient on dialysis.

LAMINAR FLOW - Streamlined flow of a viscous fluid near a solid boundary.

LEACH - Occurs when a fluid passes through a substance and dissolves away part of that substance. In water treatment, copper lead, or galvanized steel pipes should not be used after the blending valve because water can leach copper from the copper pipes, or zinc from the galvanized pipes.

LEAK TESTING - See Pressure Testing.

LEUKOCYTE - White blood corpuscle or blood cells. There are two types: granulocytes, and agranulocytes.

LIDOCAINE - A local anesthetic drug. Trade name is Xylocaine.

LOADING DOSE - A dose of medication that creates a certain level in the body. A loading dose of heparin may be given after both needles are in place, but before the treatment begins, to allow that heparin to circulate throughout the patient's body.

LOCAL INFECTION - An infection only in one specific area—such as in a blood vessel or graft and the surrounding tissues.

LOOP OF HENLE – Part of the nephron; the descending and ascending loops of the renal tubule, between the proximal convoluted tubule and the distal convoluted tubule.

LUMEN - The lumen is the inside diameter of a tube (i.e., catheter or needle) or a tubular organ (i.e., an artery or vein). In stenosis, the lumen of the vascular access becomes narrower, limiting the blood flow.

LYSE - To lyse is to dissolve. One option for treating a blood clot in a vascular access is to use a medication that will lyse the clot.

MAGNESIUM - A metallic mineral. It is found in the body as an electrolyte in the intracellular fluid; a small trace of magnesium in body fluids is essential to the function of the nervous system. (*See also: Dialysate*).

MASTER FILE OR MASTER RECORD - Summary of all reprocessing procedures, specifications, policies and procedures, training materials, manuals, and methods for reprocessing.

MATERIAL SAFETY DATA SHEET (MSDS) - Prepared and supplied by the manufacturer of the chemical, it contains information on that chemical and corrective action to take in the event of a spill or exposure.

MATTER - Anything that occupies a space, may be gaseous or solid.

MEDICARE ESRD PROGRAM - Was established by the U.S. congress in 1972. The program extended Medicare benefits to the patients with renal disease that were entitled to Social Security Benefits. The ESRD program pays for 80% of the allowable cost of dialysis treatment for eligible patients.

MEMBRANE FILTERS - Membrane filters are water treatment cartridges containing thin membranes with pores of a specified size. Membrane filters remove small particles and some solutes.

METABOLIC ACIDOSIS - A condition in which the acid/base balance of a body fluid has shifted toward acidic because there is a build-up of acid in the body. Dialysis patients commonly develop metabolic acidosis, because their kidneys no longer appropriately reabsorb bicarbonate—a blood buffer that stabilizes blood pH. For this reason, bicarbonate is usually used as a buffer for dialysate. (*See also: Bicarbonate, Buffer*).

METABOLISM - The sum of chemical processes that involve breaking down some substances and creating other substances.

METASTATIC CALCIFICATION - See Extraskeletal Calcification.

MICROALBUMINURIA - The presence of tiny amounts of albumin in the urine. This condition, measured by a simple urine test, can be an early indicator of chronic renal failure, because albumin is too large a molecule to pass through healthy glomeruli. A class of blood pressure medications called ACE inhibitors, such as catopril, has been shown to slow progression of kidney failure is diabetic patients with microalbuminuria. (*See also: Albumin*).

MICRONS - The unit of measure for filter pores. Filters with high micron sizes trap large particles and allow smaller particles to flow through. A submicron filter may be required to capture very small particles. (*See also: Filters*).

MICROORGANISMS - Living things too small to be seen without a microscope. Algae, fungi, bacteria, and viruses are types of microorganisms. Some microorganisms can cause illness if they enter the body. Bacteria are important sources of microorganism contamination for dialysis patients. (*See also: Bacteria*).

MIDDLE MOLECULES - Molecules with a molecular weight in the range of 300 to 2,000 that diffuse poorly across conventional membranes. Molecules in this range are suspected of being a cause of uremic neuropathogenicity.

MODALITY - A type of treatment such as hemodialysis, peritoneal dialysis, or transplantation.

MOLECULAR WEIGHT - A measure of the size of a molecule. Weight of a molecule attained by totaling the atomic weight of its constituent atoms. Molecular weight is measured in Daltons. Large molecules (like beta-2-microglobulin) have high molecular weights.

MOLECULAR WEIGHT CUTOFF - The solute range that can pass through a particular semipermeable membrane.

MOLECULE - The smallest complete unit of a substance that retains that substance's identity.

MORBIDITY - Illness. Morbidity sometimes measured as days of hospitalization, is used as one measure of patient outcomes.

MORTALITY - Death. Mortality is used as one measure of patient outcomes.

MYALGIA - Muscle pain.

MYOCARDIAL INFRACTION - The blockage of a heart artery, which can lead to death in part of the heart muscle. The patient may feel severe or crushing chest pain—a "heart attack". Myocardial infraction is commonly abbreviates as MI. (*See also: Arrhythmia*).

NASOGASTRIC (NG) TUBE - A tube that is inserted through the nose into the stomach. Patients who are extremely malnourished may need to be fed through the NG tube.

NEGATIVE PRESSURE - Pressure that is less than 0 mmHg, created by suction, or a vacuum. In dialysis, negative pressure is created by a pump, which pulls fluid from the blood compartment. Negative pressure plus positive pressure equals transmembrane pressure. (*See also: Positive Pressure, Transmembrane Pressure, and Ultrafiltration*).

NEOINTIMAL HYPERPLASIA - Occurs when smooth muscle cells at the venous anastomosis form extra layers of cells that fill up the graft lumen, reducing blood flow. (*See also: Anastomosis, Lumen*).

NEPHROLOGIST - A doctor who specializes in kidney disease.

NEPHROLOGY - The study of the kidneys. As a medical specialty, nephrology deals with information, care, and knowledge of kidneys. A nephrologist is a doctor of internal medicine who specializes in nephrology. A pediatrician nephrologist is a physician who specializes in the care of children and adolescents with kidney disease. A nephrology nurse has a special training in the care of people with renal failure. A nephrology technician has training in the care of people with renal failure and the technology that supports their care.

NEPHRONS - Tiny blood purification filters contained in the kidneys. Nephrons filter all of the waste products from the body, and maintain electrolyte and fluid balance. Each kidney contains approximately one million microscopic nephrons. Each nephron has its own tiny blood vessels (capillaries) that supply it with blood to be cleaned. Each nephron is made up of a glomerulus and tubules. (*See also: Glomerulus*).

NEUROPATHY - See Peripheral Neuropathy.

NKF-DOQI (NATIONAL KIDNEY FOUNDATION – DIALYSIS OUTCOMES QUALITY INITIATIVE) CLINICAL PRACTICE GUIDELINES - See Clinical Practice Guidelines.

NON-POTABLE - Not suitable for consumption (drinking).

NORMAL SALINE - A sterile salt-water solution containing 0.9% sodium chloride, equal to the concentration of sodium chloride found in the blood. In hemodialysis, normal saline is needed to prime and prepare the extracorporeal circuit, and is used for fluid replacement during the treatment.

NO TRANSFER LEVEL – Limits set by AAMI for trace metals in water used for dialysis treatment. A level low enough so that none of the substances will transfer from dialysate into the patient's blood. (i.e., lead, mercury, arsenic, silver).

NOSOCOMIAL - Means hospital acquired. The term is usually applied to infections or illnesses patients acquire during the course of their medical treatment while in the hospital or nursing home environment.

OLIGURIA – Urinary output of less than 400 cc/day; usually results in renal failure if not reversed. Seen after profuse perspiration, bleeding, diarrhea, and renal failure due to any disease. Also in retention disease of the central nervous system, shock, drug poisoning, deep coma, or hypertrophy of the prostate.

OPPORTUNISTIC ILLNESSES - Occurs when a patient's immune system is impaired, or weakened. Patients with AIDS, for example, are vulnerable to opportunistic infections because their immune systems have been compromised.

ORGAN - A part of the body having a special function. Many organs are in pairs. In such pairs, one organ may be extirpated and the remaining one can perform all necessary functions peculiar to it. One-third to two fifths of some organs may be removed without loss of function necessary to support life.

ORGANIC - Chemical substances that contain carbon.

ORGAN SYSTEM – A group of organs related to each other and performing a certain functions together (i.e., digestive system).

ORTHOSTATIC HYPOTENSION - A drop in blood pressure of 15 mmHg or more when a person rises from a sitting to standing position.

OSHA (OCCUPATIONAL SAFETY HEALTH ASSOCIATION) - A federal agency that oversees safety and health regulations for employees in the work place. Occupational exposure to blood borne pathogens (HBV, HIV). Occupational exposure to formaldehyde and other chemicals. Hazards communications (MSDS).

OSMOSIS - The movement of fluid across a semipermeable membrane from an area of lower solute concentration (like blood) to and area of high solute concentration (like dialysate) until the solute concentrations on both sides of the membrane are equal. Natural osmosis is too slow to produce enough fluid removal for hemodialysis, so fluid movement is aided with a hydraulic pressure gradient.

OSMOTIC GRADIENT - A difference in concentration of solutes on each side of a semipermeable membrane.

OSMOTIC PRESSURE - Is an osmotic gradient created by using dialysate containing substances, such as glucose, that cause fluid to move out of the blood and into the dialysate. (*See also: Dialysate, Osmosis*).

OSTEOSCLEROSIS – An abnormal increase in thickening and density of the bone.

OSTETITIS FIBROSA CYSTICA – See hyperparathyroid bone disease.

OXIDANTS – Chemicals used for disinfection in the reprocessing of dialyzers, such as bleach, renalin, hydrogen peroxide and amuchina; they combine with oxygen to breakdown cell walls killing bacteria.

OXIDIZERS - Chemicals combined with oxygen to break down cell walls. (*See also: Oxidants*).

PALPATE - To exam by touch; to feel.

PALPITATIONS - Are occasional, strong heartbeats that can be a symptom of cardiac arrhythmia.

PARATHYROID HORMONE (PTH) - A hormone produced by four parathyroid glands located in the neck. PTH is released into the bloodstream in the large amounts when the calcium levels are low—a common problem in patients with renal failure—or when levels of phosphorous in the bloodstream are high. Too much PTH can cause hyperparathyroid bone disease. The synthetic form of calcitriol is given to most dialysis patients to help them avoid bone disease. (*See also: Calcium*).

PATENCY - The state of openness or the lack of obstruction of a blood vessel or catheter. Before beginning dialysis, patency of the patient's internal access should be checked by listening for the bruit, or feeling for the thrill. (*See also: Access, Bruit, Thrill*).

PATHOGEN - An agent (such as bacteria) that causes disease in humans. (*See also: Bacteria*).

PATHOLOGY - The study of the nature of the cause of disease, which involves changes in structure and function.

PATIENT OUTCOMES - Are the results of care. Morbidity and mortality are traditionally measured outcomes, but other outcomes such as "functional status"—the ability to do usual activities (activities of daily living, or ADLs)—are gaining in importance. Successful rehabilitation is also a patient outcome.

PERICARDIAL EFFUSION - A build-up of fluid in the pericardium, or sac surrounding the heart. In severe cases, pericardial infusion can lead to cardiac tamponade, a potentially life threatening condition in which fluid pressure makes it difficult or impossible for the heart to beat.

PERICARDITIS - An inflammation of the pericardium, the membrane, or sac that surrounds the heart. Pericarditis causes low-grade fever, hypotension, and persistent pain in the center of the chest that may be relieved by sitting up and taking deep breaths. Patients who are uremic or inadequately dialyzed may be prone to pericarditis.

PERICIARDIUM - The double membranous fibroserous sac enclosing the heart and the origins of the great blood vessels. It is composed of an inner serous layer and outer fibrous layer.

PERIPHERAL - Means away from the center of the body.

PERIPHERAL NEUROPATHY - Neuropathy is nerve damage. Peripheral neuropathy includes symptoms of numbness, tingling, burning, pain and weakness in the hands and feet. In dialysis patients, neuropathy may be caused by one or more toxins retained in uremia and inadequately removed by hemodialysis. Neuropathy may also be a result of vascular access problems, which may lead to waste build-up due to inadequate dialysis. Many cases of peripheral neuropathy can be prevented or treated with adequate dialysis and adherence to diet.

PERIPHERAL VASCULAR RESISTANCE - Is a measure of the ability of blood to flow through the blood vessels. A decrease in peripheral resistance (relaxation of blood vessels) will reduce blood pressure if the heart cannot compensate. An increase in peripheral vascular resistance (narrowing of blood vessels) will increase the blood pressure.

PERITONEAL DIALYSIS (PD) - Is a type of dialysis that uses the peritoneum (a blood vessel rich sac surrounding the abdominal organs) as a semipermeable membrane. A catheter is surgically inserted into the abdominal cavity to allow sterile dialysate to fill the abdomen, dwell, and drain out. During the dwell time, wastes and excess fluid move from the blood across the peritoneum and into the dialysate by diffusion and osmosis. The peritoneal membrane in the abdomen functions in the same way as the semipermeable membrane in the dialyzer. (*See also: Dwell time*).

PERITONEUM - Is a smooth, thin layer of tissue rich in blood vessels, which covers the outside of all the abdominal organs and the inside of the abdominal walls. The peritoneum forms a closed system, somewhat like a sac, and can be used as a semipermeable membrane and the container for dialysate, in the peritoneal dialysis. (*See also: Peritoneal Dialysis*).

PERITONITIS - Is a painful infection of the peritoneum. In people on peritoneal dialysis peritonitis is a complication that can occurs when sterile technique is not properly followed during an exchange. (*See also: Peritoneal Dialysis, Sterile*).

PERMEABILITY - The quality of being permeable; capable of allowing the passage of fluids or substances in a solution. The property or state of allowing the passage of certain substances.

PERMEABLE - Means allowing substances to pass through. Cell membranes in the human body are freely permeable to water, letting fluid pass in and out. Hemodialyzer membranes have varying degrees of permeability, depending on the type of material used and the manufacturing technique; they are semipermeable.

pH - Is an expression of the hydrogen ion (acid) concentration of a solution. A solution with a pH above 7 is alkaline, or base; a solution with a pH below 7 is an acid. A solution with a pH of 7.0 is neutral. Normal body pH ranges between 7.35 and 7.45, slightly alkaline. It is important for the pH of dialysate to be within the acceptable range. Bicarbonate-buffered dialysate should have a pH of 7.2 to prevent bacterial growth and the formation of precipitation that could damage equipment. AAMI recommends that water with a pH between 6.0 and 8.0 be used to mix dialysate. (*See also: AAMI, Acid, Base, Bicarbonate*).

PHOSPHATE BINDERS - Medications that bind with phosphorous in food so the phosphorous is not absorbed into the bloodstream, but calcium can be absorbed. Phosphorous is then eliminated in the stool. Patients should take more binders with larger meals, fewer binders with small meals or snacks.

PHOSPHOROUS - A non-metallic element present in dairy products, meat, poultry, fish, nuts, peanuts, chocolate, and colas. Phosphorous is difficult to avoid in the diet, and damaged kidneys have a difficult time removing it from the blood. Too much phosphorous in the blood can cause secondary hyperparathyroidism and bone disease. Phosphorous levels are checked monthly before dialysis, and most people with renal failure take phosphate binders to control phosphorous. (*See also: Secondary Hyperparathyroidism*).

PHYSIOLOGY - The science of the function of the living organisms and its components and of the chemical and physical processes involved.

PLASTICIZER - Is a chemical that makes plastic flexible. Priming the dialyzer and blood tubing before use will help clear them of residual plasticizers. (*See also: Priming*).

PLASMA - The liquid part of the lymph and of the blood.

PLATELETS - Blood cells that promote clotting by clumping together when "activated" by signals sent by injured cells.

PNEUMOTHORAX - Is air in the chest cavity that prevents the lungs from expanding. Pneumothorax can occur during central venous catheter placement if the catheter punctures a blood vessel and passes into the space between the lungs and the chest wall.

POLYMER - A polymer is a long string of small molecules that's similar to plastic used to make dialyzer semipermeable membranes. (i.e., cellulose polymer, synthetic polymer).

POLYCYSTIC KIDNEY DISEASE (PKD) - An inherited disease that causes large, fluid-filled cysts to develop in the kidneys. The cysts can even become so large and numerous that they crowd out normal kidney tissue, which can cause kidney failure.

PORES - Pores are holes. In a semipermeable dialyzer membrane, membrane filter, or reverse osmosis unit, the size of the pores is designed to allow solutes of a certain size range to pass through, while trapping solutes that are too large to fit through.

POSITIONAL - Means affected by the patient's body position. When hemodialysis catheters are positional, blood flow can be interrupted or decreased by the patient's movement. If the patient coughs or changes position, the blood flow may improve because their catheter may move within the blood vessel.

POSITIVE PRESSURE - Is pressure greater that zero mmHg. A pressure that is greater than atmospheric pressure. In dialysis, positive pressure is created when the blood pump pushes blood through the pores in the semipermeable membrane. Positive and negative pressure together equal transmembrane pressure. (*See also: Negative Pressure, Transmembrane Pressure, Ultrafiltration*).

POSTDIALYZER PRESSURE - See Venous Pressure.

POSTPUMP ARTERIAL PRESSRUE - See Predialyzer Pressure.

POTASSIUM - A metallic element, and important electrolyte in the human body. Correct levels of potassium are needed for optimal functioning of the body's cells. (*See also: Electrolyte, Hyperkalemia, Hypokalemia*).

POTTING SOIL - Polyurethane clay-like material at both ends of the dialyzer that holds the hollow fibers open for blood to flow inside of the fiber.

PRECIPITATE - See Scale.

PREDIALYZER PRESSURE - Is the positive pressure after the blood pump and before the dialyzer. Predialyzer pressure is also called postpump pressure, or postpump arterial pressure.

PREPROCESSING - Means putting a new dialyzer through all the reprocessing steps before it is used for the first time. This process helps remove residual amounts of ETO or other substances used during manufacturing that might cause allergic or hypersensitivity reactions.

PREPUMP ARTERIAL PRESSURE - A measurement of the pressure between the patient's arterial needle site and the blood pump. Prepump arterial pressure represents the negative pressure created by the blood pump. Arterial pressure monitoring guards against excessive suction on the vascular access.

PRESSURE - A force applied to an object by something that comes in contact with an object. In the human body, blood pressure is the combination of flow or force from the heart, resistance in the blood vessels. In hemodialysis, pressure is the combination of flow from the blood pump and resistance in the dialyzer and extracorporeal circuit.

PRESSRUE GRADIENT - See Transmembrane Pressure.

PRESSURE TESTING – (Leak testing) Ensures that a dialyzer membrane is intact and no blood loss will occur during the next use. Pressure testing must be a part of the reuse process. (*See also: Reprocessing*).

PRIMING - Filling and rinsing the bloodlines and the dialyzer with a solution of normal saline. The priming solution for the dialysate compartments is dialysate. Priming is done before dialysis to remove air, disinfecting chemicals, and some plasticizing chemicals from the extracorporeal circuit and dialysate side of the dialyzer. (*See also: Dialyzer, Disinfectant, Plasticizer*).

PRIMING VOLUME - The amount of solution necessary to fill a compartment of the dialyzer before dialysis can begin.

PRODUCT WATER - Water that has been forced through a reverse osmosis membrane. (*See also: Reverse Osmosis*).

PROPORTIONING SYSTEM - A type of dialysate delivery system. Proportioning systems mix liquid concentrate with specific amounts of treated water to form dialysate and deliver it to the dialyzer. Proportioning systems are available in two types: fixed-ratio pumps and servo-controlled mechanisms. These systems use dual conductivity meters to check the mixed dialysate continuously and to support the system, should one monitor fail. (*See also: Hemodialysis Delivery System*).

PROTEINURIA – Means protein in the urine. When kidneys are damaged, protein can leak through the glomeruli into the renal tubules and into the urine. (*See also: Glomerulus, Microalbuminuria*).

PROXIMAL - Means nearest the point of attachment, center of the body or point of reference; the opposite of distal.

PROXIMAL CONVOLUTED TUBULE – Part of the nephron tubules, which lies between the Bowman's Capsule and the Loop of Henle.

PRURITUS - A severe and constant itching. Itching may develop in patients with renal failure due to dry skin or a build-up of calcium phosphate crystals in the skin. Adequate dialysis, good management of calcium phosphorous, limiting bathtub soaking time, and use of some lotions or creams can help reduce itching. Unless pruritus is relieved the patient may become exhausted from lack of sleep.

PSEUDOANEURYSM - Is a false aneurysm, a bulging pocket of blood surrounding a fistula or more commonly an ePTFE graft. Pseudoaneurysms can occur if a graft has been repeatedly punctured in the same area. (*See also: aneurysm*).

PUMP OCCLUSION - The amount of space between the rollers of the blood pump and the pump housing. The rollers of the blood pump should compress the blood tubing segment against the blood pump house enough to close the lumen completely at that point. Over occlusion produces excess pressure that may crack the tubing causing the pumping segment to rupture. If occlusion is not complete, there will be backflow of blood with each pump stroke. (*See also: Blood Pump Segment*).

PURE ULTAFILTRATION - See Isolated Ultrafiltration.

PURPURA - Bleeding under the skin, which may be a symptom of heparin overdose or platelet dysfunction. The outward manifestations and laboratory findings of primary and secondary purpura are similar. There is bleeding under the skin, with easy bruising and the development of petechiae. In the acute form there may be bleeding from any of the body orifices, such as hematuria, nosebleed, vaginal bleeding, and bleeding gums. (*See also: Heparin*).

PYROGEN - A fever producing substance such as endotoxin – a component of the outer walls of bacteria.

PYROGENIC REACTION - Are symptoms caused by pyrogens (such as endotoxins), which may include shills, fever, shaking, hypotension, vomiting, and myalgia. Dialysis patients may have pyrogenic reactions if they are exposed to improperly treated water or an endotoxin-contaminated reprocessed dialyzer. (*See also: Endotoxin*).

QUALITY ASSURANCE (QA) - A mechanism or program used by facilities to monitor, evaluate, and improve care. It is based on measuring facilities' quality of care against predetermined standards. (*See also: Clinical Practice Guidelines, Continuous Quality Improvement*).

RADIAL ARTERY - Artery located in the forearm on the thumb side of the wrist.

RADIAL PULSE – An artery in the forearm, wrist, and hand; the one usually used for taking the pulse.

RADIOCEPHALIC FISTULA - Connects the radial artery and the cephalic vein in the distal forearm to create a vascular access for hemodialysis. This is the most common type of AV fistula.

REAGENT - A material that will react in the presence of a certain chemical. Reagent strips are used to make sure all chemical residues are removed from a reprocessed dialyzer or the dialysis delivery system, or test for the presence of blood in dialysate. (*See also: Hemastix*).

RECIRCULATION - Occurs when already-dialyzed blood returning to the patient through the venous needle mixes with undialyzed blood entering the arterial needle. Blood entering the dialyzer can become diluted with blood that just left the dialyzer. This occurs as a result of retrograde flow through the vascular access segment between the arterial and venous needle sites. Recirculation greater that 15% is significant, and reduces hemodialysis adequacy. (*See also: Hemodialysis Adequacy, Retrograde*).

RECOMBINANT - Means cloned. A recombinant substance such as EPOGEN has been developed by genetic engineering techniques. (*See also: EPOGEN*).

REJECTION - Occurs when the immune system of a transplant patient attacks the transplanted organ because it is foreign to the body. The risk of rejection is reduced by matching the patient's blood type and tissue type the organ the body is less likely to recognize the organ as foreign, and by using immunosuppressant drugs to reduce the body's immune response to the transplanted organ.

REJECT WATER - The waste or reject stream that is sent to the drain along with the solutes removed by the reverse osmosis.

RENAL FAILURE - See acute renal failure, chronic renal failure.

RENAL NEUROPATHY – Disease of the nerves caused by chronic renal failure or uremia, causing symptoms such as loss of sensation (or painful sensation) in the hands or feet, muscle weakness, impaired reflexes.

RENAL OSTEODYSTROPHY - Generalized pathological changes in bone with resemblance to Osteitis Fibrosa Cystica, osteomalacia, and osteoporosis. These changes are associated with renal failure. The serum phosphorous is elevated, calcium is low or normal, and there is increased parathyroid gland activity.

RENIN - An enzyme produced by the kidney to control blood pressure. Renin splits angiostensinogen to form a pressor substance angiotensin I, which is then transformed into angiotensin II, which stimulates vasoconstriction and secretion of aldosterone.

RENIN-ANGIOSTENSIN-ALDOSTERONE SYSTEM – Helps control blood pressure in healthy individuals. Renin is an enzyme produced by kidneys during stress. Renin combines with another substance to form angiostensin, a hormone that tightens the blood vessels, raising blood pressure. (*See also: Renin*).

REPROCESSING - The process of cleaning and disinfecting dialyzers and, in some cases, bloodlines, to be used on the same patient. Done carefully, reprocessing reduces the cost of dialyzers and offers some benefits to patients. The hazardous chemicals used in reprocessing must be handled with care by staff. A number of regulations and guidelines are in place to protect patients and staff when reprocessed dialyzers are used.

RESIDUAL BLOOD VOLUME - The amount of blood remaining in the extracorporeal circuit after termination of hemodialysis treatment.

RESISTANCE - Is created by any factor that partially obstructs flow. In dialysis, there is resistance against the flow of blood in the blood vessels or in the extracorporeal circuit. Flow and resistance influence pressure.

RESISTIVITY - The measure of the forces that oppose the flow of electricity through a fluid. (*See also: Conductivity*).

RETROGRADE - Means against the direction of flow. In a fistula or graft, retrograde flow is toward the anastomosis. The arterial needle may be placed either retrograde or anterograde in the access. (*See also: Anastomosis*).

REUSE - The practice of cleaning and sterilizing a used dialyzer that is to be used again by the same patient. (*See also: Reprocessing*).

REVERSE OSMOSIS - A membrane separation process for removing solutes from a solution. A reverse osmosis unit is a cartridge containing a water pressure pump and a semipermeable membrane. The RO membrane can remove 90% to 99% of many substances, including bacteria, endotoxin, viruses, salts, particles, and dissolved organics. RO membranes are used to purify or treat the water used for hemodialysis or reprocessing. Because RO membranes are costly and delicate, other filters are used to remove particles in feed water that might damage the RO membrane.

REVERSE ULTRAFILTRATION - Moving fluid through the dialyzer membrane from the dialysate compartment into the blood compartment to remove the protein layer that occurs during treatment.

RINSE BACK - The process of using saline to flush the patient's blood back into the body after dialysis. The amount of fluid necessary to clear the dialyzer.

ROLLER PUMP - Is the most common type of blood pump. A motor turns the roller head, continuously moving blood through the extracorporeal circuit.

SAGITTAL PLANE - A vertical plane through the longitudinal axis of the trunk dividing the body into two portions, right and left.

SALICYLATE - A salt of salicylic acid (aspirin).

SALINE INFUSION LINE – A line connected to the arterial blood-tubing segment just before the blood pump, so saline can be pulled into the circuit. The saline infusion line allows saline to be given to the patient during dialysis.

SCALE – (precipitate) is solid particles that settle out of a solution (i.e., water, dialysate) and can clog pipes or damage components of the water treatment system. Hard water, which contains more minerals and salts, can form scale.

SECONDARY HYPERPARATHYROIDISM - The overproduction of parathyroid hormone (PTH) due to renal failure, which can cause bone disease. With too much PTH is the blood, calcium is withdrawn from the bones, making them weak.

SEDIMENT FILTER - See filters.

SEIZURES - Are involuntary muscle spasms and loss of consciousness. Some patients may have seizures as a dialysis side effect (severe hypotension) or an adverse reaction during dialysis, such as delivery of improperly prepared dialysate.

SELF-CARE HEMODIALYSIS - Self-care hemodialysis is a form of in-center hemodialysis in which patients perform most or all of their own care with minimal staff assistance. Self-care patients may set up their own machines, insert needles, take their own vital signs, monitor the treatment, and clean up their station after treatment. Participating in self-care at some level helps the patients regain control of their lives, and helps their rehabilitation.

SEMIPERMEABLE – Half-permeable. A membrane that will allow fluids, but not the dissolved substance to pass through it. (*See also: Membrane, Osmosis*).

SEMIPERMEABLE MEMBRANE - A semipermeable membrane is a material with submicroscopic openings or pores. In hemodialysis, the semipermeable membrane's pores allows some substances (such as water) to pass through freely, while keeping other substances (such as red blood cells) from passing through. The size of the pores of the semipermeable membrane is one of the factors that affects the efficiency of the dialysis. Solute particles larger that these pores are retained. Particles small enough to pass through the pores do so at a rate inversely proportional to their size; very small particles pass quicker than larger particles.

SEPSIS/SEPTICEMIA - A life threatening infection of the blood caused by bacteria entering the bloodstream. Septicemia is also call bacteremia or sepsis.

SEQUENTIAL ULTRAFILTRATION - See Isolated ultrafiltration.

SERUM - A serous fluid that moistens the surfaces of serous membranes. The watery portion of blood after coagulation; a fluid found when clotted blood is left standing long enough for the clot to shrink.

SHUNT - A bypass. A tube that is inserted into the body. A shunt, or cannula, was the first permanent vascular access for dialysis, developed in 1960 by doctor Belding Scribner and Dr. Wayne Quinton. A Teflon tube was used to connect a flexible length of Silastic tubing to the patient's artery and vein for dialysis, making it possible for patients with chronic renal failure to receive dialysis. Since the shunt was outside the skin, it easily became infected or clotted, and is very rarely used today.

SODIUM - An element, and an important electrolyte in the human body. Sodium influences the movement of fluid across the cell membranes between the intracellular and extracellular spaces. Sodium is present in dialysate. Some dialysate delivery systems allow the sodium concentration of the dialysate to be adjusted throughout the treatment, according to a doctor's prescription. The sodium variation has been shown to create more effective fluid removal, as well as better control of blood pressure. Too little sodium in dialysate can cause hemolysis. Too much sodium in dialysate can cause crenation. (*See also: Crenation, Electrolyte, Hemolysis, Hypernatremia, Hyponatremia*).

SODIUM MODELING - Refers to tailoring the concentration of sodium in the dialysate to fit the needs of an individual patient, according to the physician's prescription.

SOLUTE DRAG - Is the movement of solute molecules along with water through a membrane's tiny pores. Solute drag is also known as convection or convective solute transfer.

SOLUTES - Particles dissolved in fluid. Many of the substances that need to be removed from the blood of renal patients (such as urea) are solutes dissolved in the blood. Solute size in measured by molecular weight. Different semipermeable membrane materials are more or less efficient at removing solutes of a certain size. (*See also: Molecular Weight*).

SOLUTE TRANSFER – Movement of solutes across the semipermeable membrane. (*See also: Diffusion, Solute Drag*).

SOLUTION - A combination of a solvent, or fluid and a solute.

SPINAL (VERTEBRAL) CAVITY – Cavity that extends downward from the cranial cavity and is surrounded by bony vertebrae that contains the spinal cord.

SPHYMOMANOMETER - An instrument for determining arterial blood pressure indirectly. The two types are aneroid and mercury. (*See also: Blood Pressure*).

SPORE - The reproductive form of some bacteria, which are very resistant to heat. Bleach is effective against many spores. The reproductive element, produced sexually or asexually, of one of the lower organisms, such as protozoa, fungi, or algae. (*See also: Bacteria, Disinfectant, Heat Disinfection*).

STAFF ASSISTED DIALYSIS —See In-center Hemodialysis.

STANDARD PRECAUTIONS – Are infection control procedures that prevent the spread of disease by treating body fluids from all patients as if they could cause infection. Important Standard Precautions include washing hands, wearing protective clothing, avoiding needle injuries by never cutting or recapping needles, using airway equipment during mouth-to-mouth resuscitation, disposing of infectious waste properly, minimizing the handling of soiled laundry, and cleaning surfaces thoroughly. Standard Precautions combine the major features of Universal Precautions, which reduce the risk of transmitting blood borne pathogens, and Body Substance Isolation, which reduces the risks of transmitting pathogens from moist body fluids and substances.

STASIS - A state of equilibrium among opposing forces. A stoppage or diminution of flow, as of blood or another body fluid.

STORAGE - A system of conditions under which reprocessed dialyzers are kept until their next use.

STANDING ORDERS - Standing orders are orders that stay the same; they are written by the physician to meet the patients' usual treatment needs. The orders should include all aspects of the care of renal patients (i.e., blood flow rate, dialysate flow rate, dialyzer, and dialysate composition).

STEAL SYNDROME - Steal syndrome occurs when a fistula or graft "steals" too much blood away from the distal (farthest from the center of body) part of the limb. When the access is in use during dialysis, some of the patients' blood bypasses the hand or foot to pass through the extracorporeal circuit instead. The resulting loss of blood flow or ischemia, can cause tissue damage manifested by coldness, poor function, and even gangrene of the fingertips if it is not addressed promptly. (*See also: Ischemia*).

STENOSIS - The narrowing of a blood vessel. Stenosis slows the flow of blood and causes turbulence inside the vessel, setting the stage for more serious complications such as thrombosis. (*See also: Thrombosis*).

STENTS - Small expanding metal rings that can be placed inside a fistula or graft or blood vessels that the fistula or graft feeds into (e.g., internal jugular vein) to help keep the lumen from narrowing. Stents are sometimes used to treat stenosis.

STERILE - Means completely free of all living organisms (bacteria, viruses, microorganisms).

STERILE TECHNIQUE - A series of steps used to maintain a germ-free environment or space. Step in sterile technique include washing hands before touching items in sterile package, touching sterile objects only to other sterile objects, cleaning blood ports or the other patients' skin with disinfectant before inserting a needle, and discarding any sterile supplies in wet, damaged, or torn packages. Peritoneal dialysis exchanges must be done using sterile technique to prevent infection. (*See also: Peritoneal Dialysis*).

STERILIZATION - Is the destruction of bacteria with chemicals or heat.

STREPTOKINASE - Thrombolytic agent used to help remove thrombi.

SUBCLAVIAN CATHETER - A catheter placed in a subclavian vein. According to NKF-DOQI guidelines for vascular access, the subclavian vein is no longer preferred for placement of a temporary or permanent dialysis catheter. Instead, the internal jugular is preferred, because it is less likely to cause central venous stenosis. (*See also: Central Venous Stenosis, Internal Jugular Catheter*).

SUBCLAVIAN VEIN - Large vein draining the arm.

SUBCUTANEOUS - Means under the fatty layer of skin. Sometimes medications, such as Lidocaine, a local anesthetic are injected subcutaneously.

SURFACE AREA - In hemodialysis is the amount of membrane in direct contact with blood and dialysate. A larger surface area (in either hemodialysis or peritoneal dialysis) allows more diffusion. Therefore, large surface area dialyzers normally have more urea clearance. (*See also: Diffusion*).

SYNTHETIC - See artificial.

SYSTEMIC - Means affecting the entire body. For example, septicemia is a systemic infection.

SYSTOLIC - Is the pressure inside the arteries during a heartbeat. It is the top number of a blood pressure reading. (*See also: Diastolic*).

SYSTOLE - That part of the heart cycle in which the heart is in contraction. The myocardial fibers are tightening and shortening.

TEMPERATURE ALARM - An alarm that indicates the dialysate temperature is incorrect. Dialysate that is too hot can cause hemolysis. Too cool dialysate can cause patient discomfort and reduce the efficiency of the dialysis.

TEMPORARY CATHETERS - A central venous catheter that is used for short-term vascular access, for example, when a permanent access is not mature to use. According to NKF-DOQI guidelines for vascular access, the preferred site for a temporary catheter is the internal jugular (IJ) or femoral vein. Temporary catheters may be stitched or sutured into place. (*See also: Internal Jugular Catheter*).

THORACIC CAVITY - The space lying above the diaphragm and enclosed within the walls of the thorax; the space occupied by the thoracic viscera.

THRILL - Is the vibration of blood flowing through the patient's fistula or graft. It can be felt by touching a patient's access.

THROMBECTOMY - Is a surgery or a chemical treatment (i.e., with a clot dissolving medication) to remove a thrombus or clot.

THROMBOCYTE - An old term for blood platelet.

THROMBOLYSIS - The process of injecting medication to dissolve a thrombus. Thrombolysis may be followed by surgery.

THROMBOSIS - Formation of a thrombus, or blood clot, is the most common cause of access failure. Early thrombosis in a graft or fistula is usually caused by surgical problems with the anastomosis, or by twisting of the vessel or graft.

THROMBUS - A clot formed in a blood vessel or a blood passage. A clot may occur when platelets are activated by contact with damaged blood vessel walls, dialyzer materials, or turbulence inside a blood vessel. (*See also: Platelets*).

TISSUE - A group or collection of similar cells and their intracellular substance that act together in the performance of a particular function.

TOTAL CELL VOLUME - See Fiber Bundle Volume.

TOTAL PARENTERAL NUTRITION (TPN) - Is a form of intravenous feeding to provide nutrients to patients who cannot eat or absorb through their gastrointestinal tracts. Interdialytic parental nutrition (IDPN) is TPN given during dialysis.

TRANSDUCER PROTECTORS - Small plastic cones containing filters that prevent blood or fluid from entering the pressure monitors on the dialysis machine. The transducer protectors are connected to the arterial and/or venous pressure monitors, and the monitoring lines are connected to the transducer protectors.

TRANSMEMBRANE PRESSURE (TMP) - The pressure across the dialyzer membrane (blood compartment pressure minus dialysate compartment pressure). To keep dialysate fluid from moving into the bloodstream, blood compartment pressure must be equal to or greater that dialysate compartment pressure.

TRANSPLANT - To transfer tissue or an organ from one part to another as in grafting or plastic surgery. A piece of tissue or organ used in transplantation.

TRANSPLANTATION - The surgical procedure that involves taking an organ or tissue from either a cadaver or a living person and using it to replace a diseased organ or tissue.

TRANSPORT - Movement or transfer of substances in a biological system, movement across electrolytes, nutrients, and liquids across cell membranes. Transport may occur actively, passively, or with assistance of a carrier.

TRANSVERSE PLANE - Plane that divides the body into a top and bottom portion.

TREND ANALYSIS – Review of dialyzer failures and unusual occurrences with equipment and patients in the dialysis environment.

TRENDELENBERG POSITION - A body position in which the head is placed at a 45-degree incline, with legs up. This position helps to relieve hypotension. Patients with a suspected air embolism should be placed in the Trendelenburg position on their left side.

TUBULAR REABSORPTION - The process by which water and dissolved substances (glomerular filtrate) move from tubules into the blood of peritubular capillaries. Although reabsorption occurs throughout the entire length of the renal tubule, most occurs in the proximal convoluted tubule.

TWIN CATHETERS - A form of permanent, silastic, single-lumen, catheters that are used as a permanent vascular access. Each lumen of a twin catheter has a separate subcutaneous tunnel, which may reduce the risk of infection.

ULTRADIFFUSION - Sequential dialysis; separate period of fluid removal and diffusion.

ULTRAFILTER - A fine membrane filter that removes very small particles; it is the most effective water treatment component for removing endotoxin. (*See also: Endotoxin*).

ULTRAFILTRATION – Filtration caused by a pressure gradient between two sides of a porous (filtering) material. The rate of ultrafiltration depends on the transmembrane pressure (TMP) and the characteristics of the dialyzer. Ultrafiltration also occurs naturally, as in the filtration of plasma at the capillary membrane.

ULTRAFILTRATION COEFFICIENT (KUF) - See Coefficient of Ultrafiltration.

ULTRAFILTRATION RATE (UFR) - The rate at which fluid moves from the blood into the dialysate through the semipermeable membrane. This rate depends on transmembrane pressure and the characteristics of the semipermeable membrane. The ultrafiltration rate is calculated by dividing the amount of fluid removed by the number of minutes of treatment time. In ultrafiltration control or volumetric machines, dialysate inflow and outflow are exactly balanced through special pumps. (*See also: Transmembrane Pressure*).

ULTRAFILTRATE - Fluid removed from the blood.

ULTRASONOGRAPHY – A radiologic technique in which deep structures of the body are visualized by recording the reflections (echoes) of ultrasonic waves directed into the tissues.

ULTRASOUND – Mechanical radiant energy of a frequency greater than 20,000 Hz; used in medicine in the technique of ultrasonography. (*See also: Ultrasonography*).

ULTRAVIOLET (UV) LIGHT - A form of invisible radiation that can destroy microorganisms by altering their DNA (genetic material) so they cannot multiply. Some microorganisms are more sensitive than others to the effects of UV light. Ultraviolet light uses a mercury vapor lamp that emits light at a specific wavelength, housed inside a quartz sleeve. Feed water flows over the quartz sleeve. Feed water flows over the quartz material and is exposed to the UV light. (*See also: Feed Water, Microorganisms*).

UNIVERSAL PRECATUIONS - See Standard Precautions.

UREA - The chief nitrogenous component of urine. The end product of protein metabolism. The diamide of carbonic acid, a crystalline solid having the formula CH_4N_2O; found in blood, lymph and urine.

UREA KINETIC MODLEING – A mathematical calculation of the changes in patients blood urea level during a dialysis treatment. UKM is used to determine whether a patient is receiving adequate dialysis. UKM can also help a physician predict the required time on dialysis, and assess a patient's protein catabolic rate to better meet the patient's dialysis and nutritional needs. The results of UKM are described as Kt/V, in which K is the dialyzer urea clearance in ml/min, t is the length of dialysis in minutes, and V is the volume of blood in which the urea is distributed. NKF-DOQI guidelines for hemodialysis adequacy recommend a minimum delivered Kt/V of 1.2 (prescribed Kt/V of 1.3) for adequate dialysis. BUN levels must be drawn using the slow flow or stop pump technique to ensure accuracy of the Kt/V result. (*See also: Hemodialysis Adequacy*).

UREA REDUCTION RATIO (URR) - The simplest method for estimating the delivered dose of dialysis, but it does not provide all the information needed to prescribe a dialysis treatment. BUN levels are measured before and after treatment, and the difference indicates how much urea was removed during dialysis, as a percentage of urea reduction. NKF-DOQI guidelines for hemodialysis adequacy recommend a minimum delivered URR of 65% (prescribed URR of 70%) for adequate dialysis. BUN levels must be drawn using the slow flow or stop pump technique to ensure accuracy of the URR result. (*See also: Hemodialysis Adequacy*).

UREMIA - A build-up of wastes in the blood that occurs in the last stage of kidney failure or in patients who are not receiving adequate dialysis, and more dialysis is needed. (*See also: Hemodialysis Adequacy*).

URETER - Tubes that connect each kidney to the bladder in order to carry urine out of the body.

URINE - An end product of metabolism not needed by the body that is excreted by the kidneys.

VASCULAR ACCESS - A means of repeatedly gaining entry to the patient's blood stream for hemodialysis. A vascular access must permit high enough blood flow rates to ensure effective dialysis. This is accomplished in one of three ways: by surgically connecting a patient's artery and vein to form an arteriovenous fistula, by connecting a patient's artery and vein with a piece of artificial vein (a graft), or by using a plastic tube, or catheter. The vascular access is the patient's lifeline; great care must be taken to protect it through good needle insertion technique and needle site rotation.

VASOCONSTRICTION - The decrease in the caliber of blood vessels or narrowing of the blood vessels.

VASODIALTATION - Dilation or widening of the blood vessels, small arteries and arterioles.

VENIPUNCTURE - Inserting a needle into a blood vessel. Skilled and gentle venipuncture prolongs the life of a patient's access, and enhances patient comfort. Proper venipuncture also helps ensure that the patient will receive a good dialysis treatment. It is also important to rotate venipuncture sites to avoid causing aneurysms or pseudoaneurysms to form the in patient's access. (*See also: Aneurysms, Pseudoaneurysms*).

VENOUS HYPERTENSION - A condition caused by stenosis where the venous pressure equalizes with arterial pressure causing swelling in the hand especially the thumb.

VENOUS PRESSURE - The measurement of the extracorporeal blood circuit pressure after the dialyzer and before the blood re-enters the patient's body. It may also be called post dialyzer pressure.

VENOUS PRESSURE HIGH/LOW ALARM - An alarm that monitors pressure from the monitoring site (venous chamber) to the patient's venous puncture site.

VENTRAL CAVITY - The cavity that is located toward the front part of the body. It is divided by the diaphragm into the upper thoracic cavity and the lower abdominopelvic cavity.

VIRUSES - Microorganisms that must obtain energy and food from other living cells. Many human diseases, such as the common cold, measles, polio, and HIV, are caused by viruses. Although extremely small, viruses are too large to cross an intact dialyzer membrane. However, if the membrane is damaged, any viruses contained in the dialysis water could contaminate the patient's blood. Viruses can be destroyed by various chemicals.

VOLUMETRIC - Means volume-measuring. Most dialysate delivery systems use volumetric fluid-balancing systems that compare the volume of dialysate entering and leaving the dialyzer. With volumetric control, the delivery system can be programmed to remove precisely the prescribed amount of fluid, delivering an exact prescription for ultrafiltration.

WATER SOFTENER - A component used in the water treatment system to reduce the concentration of calcium and magnesium in water that form scale. Water softeners work by a process of ion exchange. Ions of calcium and magnesium are removed from the water by a bed of electrically charged resin beads and traded for sodium ions, which form sodium chloride.

XYLOCAINE - The trade name for Lidocaine Hydrochloride.

Appendices

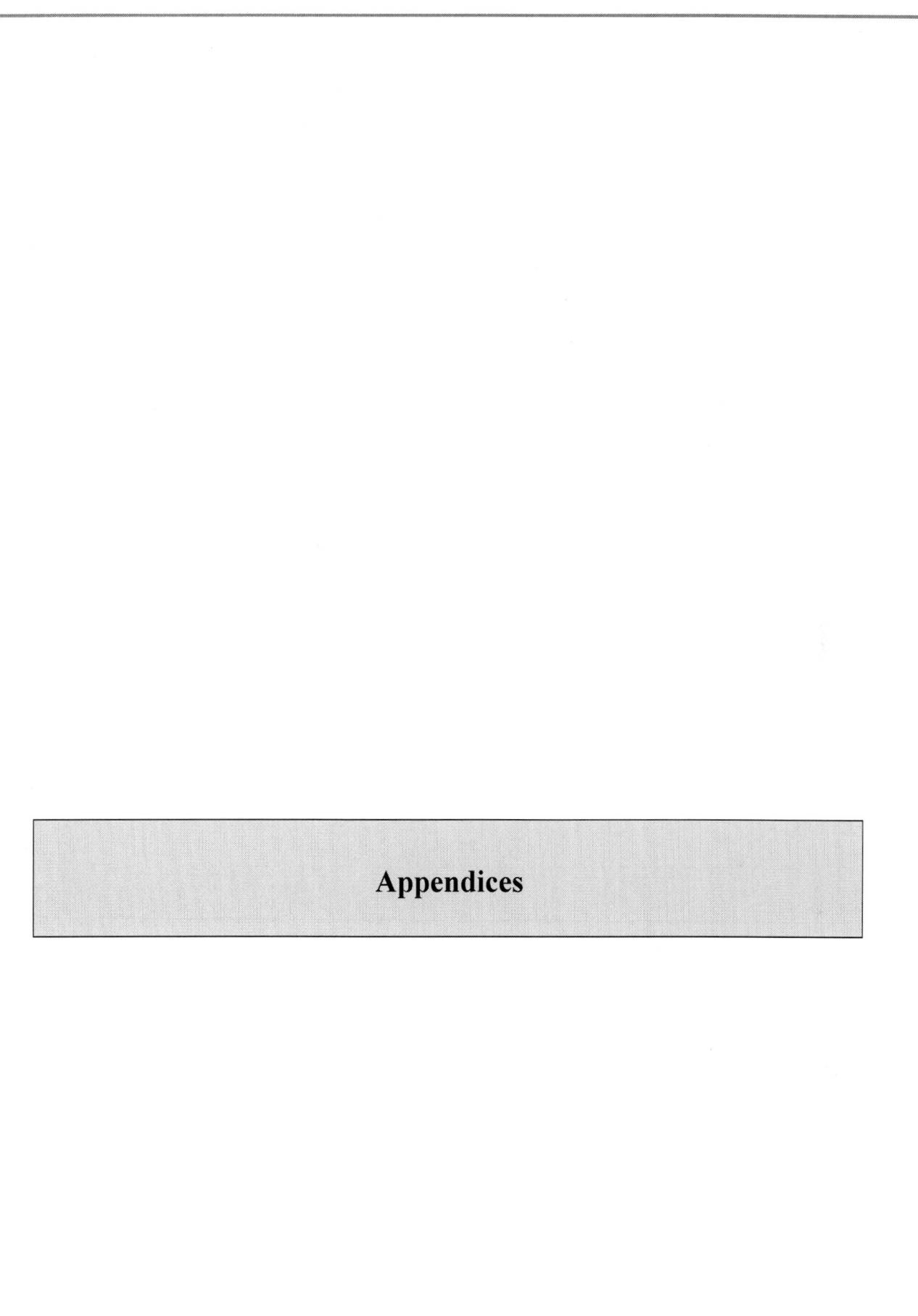

Access Options – Pros and Cons

AV Fistula

PROS	CONS
• Best overall performance • Considered the best vascular access • Less chance of infection than other types of accesses • Tend to last many years • Predictable performance • Increased blood flow	• Visible on the forearm • May take a while to develop • May require temporary access while fistula matures • Not feasible for all patients due to other medical conditions • Bleeding after the needles are removed • Fistulas may fail to mature

Grafts

PROS	CONS
• Can be readily implanted • Predictable performance • Can be used faster than AV fistula	• Increased potential for clotting • Increased potential for infection • Does not usually last as long as a fistula

Catheters

PROS	CONS
<ul><li>Dialysis can be performed immediately</li><li>Readily inserted with an outpatient procedure</li><li>Easy removal and replacement</li><li>Avoids needlesticks</li></ul>	<ul><li>Not ideal as a permanent access</li><li>High infection rates</li><li>Difficult to obtain sufficient blood flow to allow for adequate toxin removal</li><li>May cause narrowed veins</li><li>Swimming and bathing is not recommended</li></ul>

Subcutaneous Devices

PROS	CONS
<ul><li>Hemodialysis treatments can begin immediately</li><li>Allows high flow rates</li><li>Discreet and covered with clothing</li><li>Can be used for much longer periods than most temporary accesses</li><li>Needle locks into place and allows for more flexibility during dialysis</li><li>Decreased clotting</li><li>Patients may swim and bathe</li></ul>	<ul><li>Requires surgical procedure for placement under the skin</li><li>Cannot be placed in patients lacking adequate tissue</li><li>Temporary access</li><li>Requires needles</li><li>May not be available at all facilities</li><li>Healthcare professional may have limited experience using this device as it is newly available</li><li>Increased potential for infection</li></ul>

Table of commonly used equivalent values

Metric Weight/Volume

1kg = 1,000 Gm
1 Gm = 1,000 mg
1 mg = 1,000 mcg
1 mcg = 0.001 mg
1 Liter = 1,000 ml

Weights

1 oz = 30 Gm
1 Gm = 15 Grains
1 Grain = 60 mg
0.6 mg = 1/100 Grain
0.4 mg = 1/150 Grain
0.3 mg = 1/200 Grain

1 Kg = 2.2 lbs

Volume

1 quart = 960 ml
4 fl oz = 120 ml
1 fl oz = 30 ml
1 tsp = 5 ml (approximately)
1 tbs = 15 ml (approximately)
2 tbs = 30 ml (approximately)

Viral Hepatitis Overview

Type of Hepatitis	A	B	C	D	E
Source of virus	Feces	Blood/blood derived body fluids	Blood/blood derived body fluids	Blood/blood derived body fluids	Feces
Route of transmission	Fecal-oral	Percutaneous Permucosal	Percutaneous Permucosal	Percutaneous Permucosal	Fecal-oral
Chronic infection	No	Yes	Yes	Yes	No
Prevention	Pre-/post-exposure immunization	Pre-/post-exposure immunization	Blood donor screening Risk behavior modification	Pre-/post exposure immunization. Risk behavior modification	Ensure safe drinking water

Liver Function Tests

Specific Test	Normal Adult Value Ranges	Why Values Increase	Why Values Decrease
Alamine Aminotransferase (ALT)	5-35 International Units (IU)/Liter	Hepatitis, cirrhosis, liver Tumor, hepatotoxic drugs, cholestais	N/A
Aspartate Aminotransferase (AST)	5-40 IU/Liter	Myocardial infarction (MI), hepatitis, cirrhosis, acute pancreatitis, skeletal muscle trauma, liver tumor, primary muscle diseases (myopathy)	Diabetic ketoacidosis, pregnancy
Gammaglutamyl Transferase (GGT)	5-38 IU/Liter	Hepatitis, cirrhosis, liver tumor, cholestasis, alcohol ingestion, aftermath of MI	N/A
Lactate Dehydrogenase (LDH)	48-115 IU/Liter	MI, pulmonary infection, hepatitis, hemolytic anemia, pancreatitis, muscular dystrophy	N/A
Alkaline Phosphatase	30-85 IU/Liter	Cirrhosis, rheumatoid arthritis, biliary obstruction, liver tumor, hyperparathyrodism	Malnutrition, pernicious anemia, hypothyroidism
Serum Ammonia	35-65 mcg/dl	Hepatic disease, renal failure, Reye's syndrome, hepatic encephalopathy or coma	Malignant hypertension
Total Bili Direct Bili Indirect Bili	0.1-1.0 mg/dl 0.1-0.3 mg/dl 0.2-0.8 mg/dl	Cirrhosis, hepatitis, hemolytic anemia, bile duct obstruction, transfusion reaction	N/A
Serum Albumin	3.5-5.0 gm/dl	N/A	Liver disease, Crohn's disease, glomerulonephritis (GN), ascites, burns, malnutrition, lupus
Prothrombin Time	11.0-12.5 seconds	Cirrhosis, hepatitis, vitamin K deficiency, salicylate intoxication, bile duct obstruction, intake of Coumadin, disseminated intravascular coagulation (DIC)	N/A
Activated Partial Thromboplastin Time (APTT)	60-70 seconds	Clotting factor deficiencies, vitamin K deficiency, leukemia, DIC, heparin, hemophilia	N/A
Cholesterol	120-200 mg/dl	Hyperlipidimia, hypothyroidism, uncontrolled diabetes mellitus (DM), MI, hypertension, biliary cirrhosis, atherosclerosis	Malabsorption syndrome, malnutrition, hyperthyroidism, anemia, sepsis, liver disease

Formulas

Urea Reduction Ratio (URR)

$$\frac{Pre - Post}{Pre} \times 100 =$$

(65% is recommended by national guidelines)

Kt/V (Daugitdas Formula)

$$\frac{Post}{Pre} - 0.03 - \frac{UF \times Vol.\ In\ Kg}{Post\ Wt} = Natural\ Log$$

(1.2 is recommended by national guidelines)

Glomerular Filtration Rate (GFR)

$$\frac{(140 - Age) \times Wt.\ In\ Kg}{72 \times Creatinine} = GFR$$

Essential Terms of Direction and Movement

Abduction – Draws away from midline.

Adduction – Draws toward the midline.

Anterior or Ventral – Situated before or in front of.

Distal – Farther from the root.

Dorsal or Posterior – Toward the rear, back; also back of hand and top of foot.

Extension – Straightening.

External – Outside.

Frontal or Coronal – Vertical; at right angles to sagittal; divides body into anterior and posterior parts.

Horizontal – At right angles to vertical.

Inferior – Lower, farther from crown of head.

Internal – Inside.

Inverted – Turned inward.

Lateral – Farther from the midline.

Longitudinal – Refers to long axis.

Medial – Nearer to midline.

Median – Midway, being in the middle.

Midline – Divides body into right and left side.

Palmar – Palm side of the hand.

Plantar – Sole side of the foot.

Posterior or Dorsal – Rear or back.

Prone – Forearm and hand turned palm side down.

Proximal – Nearer to limb root.

Sagittal – Vertical plane or section dividing body into right and left portions.

Superficial – Nearer to surface.

Superior – Upper, nearer to crown of head.

Supine – Forearm and hand turned palm side up.

Ventral or Anterior – Situated before or in front of.

Vertical – Refers to long axis in erect position.

Related Web Sites

Dialysis Online! Message Boards:
www.be.net/~brumley/renal/index/html

Early Renal (Disease) Handbook
www.nephron.com/fkgframeset.html

Early Kidney Disease website for patients:
www.kidneydirections.com
by Baxter healthcare Corporation

E-Neph (website for journal Dialysis and Transplantation):
www.eneph.com

Polycystic kidney disease:
www.pkdcure.org

Health Care Financing Administration (HCFA):
www.hcfa.gov

Hypertension, Dialysis, and Clinical Nephrology (HDCN):
www.medtext.com/bdcn.htm

National Institute of Diabetes & Digestive & Kidney Disease (NIDDK):
www.niddk.nih.gov

National Transplant Assistance Fund (NTAF):
www.transplantfund.org

The Nephron Information Center:
www.nephron.com

Renalnet:
www.renalnet.com

Renal Rehabilitation Life Option Council:
www.lifeoptions.org

TransWeb (transplantation and donation information):
www.transweb.org

United Network for Organ Sharing (UNOS):
www.unos.org

U.S. Renal Data System (USRDS):
www.med.umich.edu/usrds

Diabetes

American Diabetes Association:
www.diabetes.com

American Diabetes Association (basic article on kidney disease and diabetes):
http://www.diabetes.org/ada/c70f.asp

DiabeticNet:
http://www.diabeticnet.com/articles/kidney.htm

OTHER SITES

References

Brenner, B. - **The Kidney** – Eight Edition, W.B. Saunders Company, Philadelpia, 2007

Daugirdas, J.T., Blake, P.G., Ing, T.S. - **Handbook of Dialysis.** Lippincott Williams and Wilkins, Philadelphia, 4th edition, 2006.

Henrich, W.L. - **Principles and Practice of Dialysis.** Lippincott Williams & Wilkins, Philadelphia, 4th edition, 2009.

Kallenbach, J. Z. - **Review of Hemodialysis for Nurses and Dialysis Personnel.** Mosby, St. Louis, Missouri, 8th edition, 2011.

Kellum, J., Bellomo, R., Ronco, C. - **Continuous Renal Replacement Therapy (Pittsburgh Critical Care Medicine).** Oxford University Press, New York, 1 edition, 2009.

Massry, S., Glassock, R. – **Textbook of Nephrology** – Fourth Edition, Lippincott Williams & Wilkins, Philadelphia, 2001.

McBride, P. – **Genesis of the Artificial Kidney** – Travenol Laboratories, 1979.

Nahas, M.E., Levin, A. - **Chronic Kidney Disease: A practical guide to understanding and management.** Oxford University Press, New York, 1 edition, 2010.

Ronco, C., Dell'Aquila, R., Rodighhiero, M.P. – **Peritoneal Dialysis a Clinical Update** – Karger, New York, 2008.

Ronco, C., La Greca, G. – **Hemodialysis Technology** – Karger, New York, 2002.

Ronco, C., Rosner, M. H. – **Hemodialysis: New Methods and Future Technology (Contributions to Nephrology**) – Karger, 1st edition, 2011.

Schrier, R.W. - **Renal and Electrolyte Disorders.** Lippincott Williams & Wilkins; 7th edition, Philadelphia , 2010.

Van Leeuvwen, M., Poelhuis-Leth, J. - **Davis's Comprehensive Handbook of Laboratory and Diagnostic Tests With Nursing Implications**. F.A. Davis, Philadelphia, 2009.

Suggestions

If you have suggestions for this book please send them to:

Medical West Publishing
P.O. Box 22
West Covina, CA 91793
USA

Or you can e-mail us at:

mwp@medicalwestpublishing.net

Practice Questions

1. A nephron is made up of:
    a. A glomerulus and a tubule
    b. The nephrons and a capsule
    c. The loop of Henle and the capillary ball
    d. The bladder and ureter

2. The functional unit of the kidney, or the structure in the kidney that does the work, is the:
    a. Medulla
    b. Cortez
    c. Calyx
    d. Nephron

3. Diffusion is movement of particles:
    a. By filtration through a biocompatible membrane
    b. From an area of higher concentration to an area of lower concentration
    c. Into a vacuum created when fluids are forced through a membrane
    d. Into a space created by solutions moving in countercurrent flows

4. Name the two compartments of the dialyzer:
    a. Conventional and high flux
    b. Convection and adsorption
    c. Blood and dialysate
    d. Hollow fiber and flat plate

5. Muscle cramps are primarily caused by the shifting concentrations of this ion during hemodialysis:
    a. Phosphorus
    b. Potassium
    c. Magnesium
    d. Sodium

6. Chloramine exposure in hemodialysis can cause:
    a. Bleeding
    b. Hypernatremia
    c. Hemolysis
    d. Pericarditis

Answer Key

1. A
2. D
3. B
4. C
5. D
6. C

NOTES

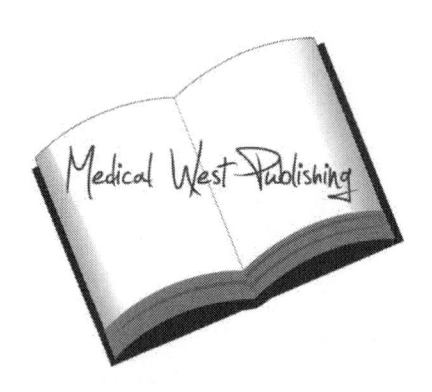

Medical West Publishing

medicalwestpublishing.net

P.O. Box 22
West Covina, California
USA
91793

Printed in Great Britain
by Amazon.co.uk, Ltd.,
Marston Gate.